D1234797

Hypertension

Guest Editor

MAHBOOB RAHMAN, MD

CLINICS IN GERIATRIC MEDICINE

www.geriatric.theclinics.com

May 2009 • Volume 25 • Number 2

SAUNDERS an imprint of ELSEVIER, Inc.

W.B. SAUNDERS COMPANY
A Division of Elsevier Inc.

1600 John F. Kennedy Blvd., Suite 1800. Philadelphia, Pennsylvania 19103-2899

http://www.theclinics.com

CLINICS IN GERIATRIC MEDICINE Volume 25, Number 2
May 2009 ISSN 0749–0690, ISBN-13: 978-1-4377-0481-5, ISBN-10: 1-4377-0481-6

Editor: Yonah Korngold

Clinics in Geriatric Medicine (ISSN 0749-0690) is published quarterly by Elsevier Inc., 360 Park Avenue South, New York, NY 10010-1710. Months of issue are February, May, August, and November. Business and Editorial Offices: 1600 John F. Kennedy Blvd., Suite 1800, Philadelphia, PA 191023-2899. Customer Service Office: 6277 Sea Harbor Drive, Orlando, FL 32887-4800. Periodicals postage paid at New York, NY, and additional mailing offices. Subscription prices is $208.00 per year (US individuals), $353.00 per year (US institutions), $271.00 per year (Canadian individuals), $440.00 per year (Canadian institutions), $288.00 per year (foreign individuals) and $440.00 per year (foreign institutions). Foreign air speed delivery is included in all *Clinics* subscription prices. All prices are subject to change without notice. POSTMASTER: Send address changes to *Clinics in Geriatric Medicine,* Elsevier Periodicals Customer Service, 11830 Westline Industrial Drive, St. Louis, MO 63146. **Customer Service: 1-800-654-2452 (US). From outside the United States, call 1-314-453-7041. Fax: 1-314-453-5170. E-mail: journalscustomerservice-usa@elsevier.com (for print support) or journalsonlinesupport-usa@elsevier.com (for online support).**

Reprints. For copies of 100 or more, of articles in this publication, please contact the Commercial Reprints Department, Elsevier Inc., 360 Park Avenue South, New York, New York 10010-1710. Tel.: (212) 633-3812; Fax: (212) 462-1935, email: reprints@elsevier.com.

Clinics in Geriatric Medicine is covered in *MEDLINE/PubMed (Index Medicus), EMBASE/Excerpta Medica, Current Contents/Clinical Medicine (CC/CM),* and the *Cumulative Index to Nursing & Allied Health Literature.*

Printed in the United States of America.

Contributors

GUEST EDITOR

MAHBOOB RAHMAN, MD
Associate Professor of Medicine, Division of Nephrology and Hypertension, Case Western Reserve University, University Hospitals Case Medical Center, Louis Stokes Cleveland VA Medical Center, Cleveland, Ohio

AUTHORS

DANIELLE COONEY, DPharm, BC-ADM
Clinical Pharmacy Specialist, Ambulatory Care and Renal, Department of Pharmacy, Louis Stokes Veterans Affairs Medical Center, Cleveland, Ohio

MARY V. CORRIGAN, MD
Assistant Professor, Department of Family Practice, Case Western Reserve University School of Medicine; Geriatric Fellowship Director, Section of Geriatrics, MetroHealth System, Senior Health and Wellness Center, Old Brooklyn Campus, Cleveland, Ohio

MARY ANN LIM, MD
Nephrology Fellow, Renal Electrolyte and Hypertension Division, Department of Medicine, Hospital of the University of Pennsylvania, Philadelphia, Pennsylvania

DONALD M. LLOYD-JONES, MD, ScM
Department of Medicine, The Bluhm Cardiovascular Institute; Department of Preventive Medicine, Feinberg School of Medicine, Northwestern University, Chicago, Illinois

MAHA A. MOHAMED, MD
Nephrology Fellow, Division of Nephrology, Department of Medicine, University of Maryland School of Medicine, Baltimore, Maryland

WILLIAM J. MOSLEY II, MD
Department of Medicine, The Bluhm Cardiovascular Institute, Feinberg School of Medicine, Northwestern University, Chicago, Illinois

THOMAS OLABODE OBISESAN, MD, MPH
Professor of Geriatric Medicine, Chief, Division of Geriatrics, Department of Medicine, Howard University Hospital, Washington, DC

APARNA PADIYAR, MD
Division of Nephrology and Hypertension, Department of Medicine, Case Western Reserve University, University Hospitals Case Medical Center, Cleveland, Ohio

MURALIDHAR PALLAKI, MD
Assistant Professor, Case Western Reserve University School of Medicine; Director of Geriatric Evaluation and Management Unit and Geriatric Clinics, Section of Geriatrics, Louis Stokes Veterans Affairs Medical Center, Cleveland, Ohio

KRISTINA PASCUZZI, DPharm, BCPS
Clinical Pharmacy Specialist, Ambulatory Care, Department of Pharmacy, Louis Stokes
Veterans Affairs Medical Center, Cleveland, Ohio

MOHAMMED A. RAFEY, MD, MS
Associate Staff, Department of Nephrology and Hypertension, Glickman Urological
and Kidney Institute, Cleveland Clinic Foundation, Cleveland, Ohio

ARASH RASHIDI, MD
Department of Medicine, Case Western Reserve University; and North Ohio Heart Center
and Ohio Medical Group, Cleveland, Ohio

RAYMOND R. TOWNSEND, MD
Director, Hypertension Program, Hospital of the University of Pennsylvania; Professor
of Medicine, Renal Electrolyte and Hypertension Division, Department of Medicine,
Hospital of the University of Pennsylvania, Philadelphia, Pennsylvania

MATTHEW R. WEIR, MD
Professor, Division of Nephrology, Department of Medicine, University of Maryland
School of Medicine, Baltimore, Maryland

JACKSON T. WRIGHT, Jr, MD, PhD
Professor of Medicine, Director, Clinical Hypertension Program, Program Director,
William T. Dahms Clinical Research Unit, Case Western Reserve University, Cleveland,
Ohio

Contents

Hypertension is clearly associated with cardiovascular disease (CVD) and death. With age, the incidence of hypertension increases, making it imperative that we understand the pathophysiology and treatment of hypertension, especially in the elderly. Data regarding individuals older than 80 years are emerging, with more attention being given to patterns and treatment of hypertension in the elderly. Thus far, we have done a poor job with treating hypertension; this is due to multiple factors, including a reluctance of physicians to treat hypertension in the elderly because of concern of causing harm. In this article, the author's discuss the history and pathophysiology of hypertension, hypertension population studies, and hypertension treatment studies with a focus on the elderly. The author's findings both justify and encourage antihypertensive treatment in all hypertensive adults.

The loss of arterial compliance as a result of the aging of human vasculature is thought to contribute to the age dependent rise in isolated systolic hypertension, and is an independent predictor of all cause mortality and cardiovascular outcomes. In this article, the author's we begin by providing a brief historical perspective of the study of the pulse wave. The author's then review the physiology of the normal arterial system, the effects of aging on the arterial system and the different measures of arterial stiffness. Finally, the author's review the different studies that look at arterial stiffness in the elderly, its impact on hypertension and cardiovascular outcome, and what is currently known on how to prevent vascular stiffness.

The geriatric population is growing in number and along with it, the prevalence of hypertension (HTN). The elderly have a unique set of characteristics that must be taken into account when treating this condition. Not only is it widespread, but its consequences, mainly cardiovascular and cerebrovascular, are devastating. Because the elderly have multiple comorbid concomitant conditions, the practitioner must be cognizant of polypharmacy and resistant HTN and prescribe in a safe fashion conducive to compliance and efficacy. Treatment in even the oldest old is indicated. Function and quality of life should be the driving principles when managing the elderly, be they in the ambulatory or long-term care setting.

Nonpharmacologic management of hypertension is all too often overlooked in the elderly. The Dietary Approaches to Stop Hypertension (DASH) diet, weight loss, physical activity, moderation of alcohol, and salt restriction, particularly when used in combination, are effective strategies to help control hypertension and reduce overall cardiovascular risk. Behavioral modification should form the cornerstone of hypertension treatment in the elderly.

Polypharmacy is highly prevalent in the elderly due to an increased number of co-morbid disease states that accompany aging. Hypertension is one common disease that can be challenging to treat in the elderly due to the body's physiologic changes, potential risks for side effects, medication interactions, and decreased medication adherence. A thorough medication assessment for each patient is essential when determining pharmacotherapeutic options in the elderly.

There is strong evidence supporting the benefit of antihypertensive treatment in older patients. Blood pressure goal and drug selection in the elderly is similar to that in younger populations, but there are a few special considerations in these patients. A number of studies have been conducted to determine the drugs or drug classes most effective for reducing cardiovascular complications in older patients with hypertension. This article reviews the evidence for drug treatment in this population.

The efficacy and safety of rennin angiotensin system (RAS) inhibition for lowering blood pressure in older populations has been demonstrated in a number of clinical trials. Whether a patient's age influences the overall ability of these drugs to lower blood pressure and protect against progress of cardiovascular and kidney disease has been the focus of few clinical trials. Herein, the author's review the mechanism of action of the renin angiotensin cascade and then discuss the clinical evidence surrounding the use of RAS-blocking drugs in the older population.

> Cumulative evidence implicates hypertension in the pathogenesis of Alzheimer disease. Although it may not presently be possible to completely differentiate the effects of treatment and control of hypertension itself from those of the medication used to achieve such treatment goals, efforts directed at the treatment and control of hypertension can have significant public health impact.

> Resistant hypertension is more prevalent in the elderly population. Current data clearly shows the benefit of blood pressure control in older individuals. It is important to first differentiate pseudoresistance from true resistant and institute appropriate therapy. In those patients with resistant hypertension without an identifiable cause, non invasive measurement of hemodynamic profile is an important option to achieve meet blood pressure goals.

Preface

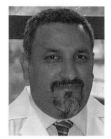

Mahboob Rahman, MD
Guest Editor

Hypertension affects more than 65 million individuals in the United States. Given the aging population, this is particularly challenging in the elderly patient; data from the Framingham study indicate that the lifetime probability of developing hypertension in the elderly is over 90%. Management of hypertension in elderly patients is a part of daily clinical practice for many primary care physicians and geriatric specialists. Therefore, this issue focusing on hypertension in the elderly is timely, and it is intended to provide the practicing clinician with a thorough update in this important area.

Several aspects of hypertension are unique in elderly patients; these are discussed in detail in this issue by authors who are experts in their areas. Drs. Mosley and Lloyd-Jones set the stage by describing the epidemiology of hypertension in the growing elderly population. Drs. Lim and Townsend illustrate the importance of arterial stiffness in the pathophysiology and management of hypertension in this population. Drs. Corrigan and Pallaki provide a thorough overview of the approach to management of hypertension, and Dr. Padiyar emphasizes the importance of lifestyle modification as an adjunctive measure to improve blood pressure control. Many elderly patients take multiple medications for a variety of medical conditions; in addition, the metabolism of drugs is often altered. Drs. Pascuzzi and Cooney provide an important review on the topic of pharmacokinetics of antihypertensive drugs in the elderly, and highlight the need to be alert to the possibility of drug interactions. Drs. Rashidi and Wright review the clinical trial literature with regard to choice of antihypertensive drug therapy in the elderly, and Drs. Mohamed and Weir focus on the risk and benefits of ACE inhibitors in this population. Dr. Obisesan highlights the growing body of knowledge showing the link between hypertension and cognitive function; this is an area that is likely to be the focus of intense research in the future. Finally, Dr. Rafey outlines a systematic approach for the elderly patient with resistant hypertension.

Clin Geriatr Med 25 (2009) ix–x
doi:10.1016/j.cger.2009.03.003
0749-0690/09/$ – see front matter © 2009 Elsevier Inc. All rights reserved.

geriatric.theclinics.com

We hope that this issue serves as a resource for practicing clinicians who are taking care of elderly patients, and that it stimulates discussion about the need for further research in this important area.

Mahboob Rahman, MD
Division of Nephrology and Hypertension
Case Western Reserve University
University Hospitals Case Medical Center
Louis Stokes Cleveland VA Medical Center
11100 Euclid Avenue
Celveland, OH 44106, USA

E-mail address:
mahboob.rahman@uhhospitals.org

Epidemiology of Hypertension in the Elderly

William J. Mosley II, MD[a], Donald M. Lloyd-Jones, MD, ScM[a,b],*

KEYWORDS
- Elderly • Hypertension • Blood pressure • J-curve
- Pulse pressure • Treatment

As our population ages, the importance of CVD as the leading cause of death in adults becomes increasingly clear.[1] One major reason for this trend is the patterns of blood pressure changes and increasing hypertension prevalence with age. Hypertension is a major risk for CVD, increasing risk in a graded fashion for total mortality, CVD mortality, coronary heart disease (CHD) mortality, myocardial infarction (MI), congestive heart failure (CHF), left ventricular hypertrophy, atrial fibrillation, stroke/transient ischemic attack, peripheral vascular disease, and renal failure. From 2001 to 2004, the prevalence of hypertension, defined as elevated blood pressure or taking antihypertensive medication, was 36% in US adult men and 35% in women aged 24 to 65 years, compared with 67% of men and 82% of women older than 75 years.[1] The prevalence nearly doubles in older Americans, with the vast majority having hypertension! In fact, data from the Framingham Heart Study, a long-standing study of CVD epidemiology, in men and women free of hypertension at 55 years indicate that the remaining lifetime risks for development of hypertension through 80 years are 93% and 91%, respectively.[2] In other words, more than 90% of individuals who are free of hypertension at 65 years will develop it during their remaining lifespan. Data regarding individuals older than 80 years are emerging, with more attention being given to patterns and treatment of hypertension in the elderly. The large burden of cardiovascular mortality in the elderly, coupled with the causal relationship of hypertension, highlights the importance of understanding the hemodynamics of blood pressure with age, the predictive value of blood pressure parameters for CVD events, blood pressure goals, and how aggressively the elderly should be treated.

[a] Department of Medicine, The Bluhm Cardiovascular Institute, Feinberg School Medicine, Northwestern University, 711 Austin St. #202, Evanston, IL 60202, USA
[b] Department of Preventive Medicine, Feinberg School of Medicine, Northwestern University, 680 N. Lake Shore Drive, Suite 1102, Chicago, IL 60611, USA
* Corresponding author. Department of Preventive Medicine, Feinberg School of Medicine, Northwestern University, 680 N. Lake Shore Drive, Suite 1102, Chicago, IL 60611.
E-mail address: dlj@northwestern.edu (D.M. Lloyd-Jones).

Clin Geriatr Med 25 (2009) 179–189
doi:10.1016/j.cger.2009.01.002
0749-0690/09/$ – see front matter © 2009 Elsevier Inc. All rights reserved.

geriatric.theclinics.com

HEMODYNAMIC PATTERNS OF BLOOD PRESSURE WITH AGE

The hemodynamic patterns of blood pressure changes with age were demonstrated by Franklin and colleagues[3] using data from the Framingham Heart Study and more recently using data from the National Health and Nutrition Examination Survey (NHANES III)[4] analysis in middle-aged and older adults in the United States. In the Framingham study, adult participants were separated into four groups according to systolic blood pressure (SBP)— less than 120 mm Hg, 120 to 139 mm Hg, 140 to 159 mm Hg, and more than 160 mm Hg measured at a single examination cycle in middle age. Arterial blood pressure components were then tracked backward from prior examinations and forward through later examinations and plotted across age—30 to 84 years. SBP increased linearly with age in all four groups, whereas diastolic blood pressure (DBP) increased up to 50 years, plateaued, but then declined after 60 years. As expected, with falling DBP and rising SBP, pulse pressure (PP) rose steeply after 60 years. The calculated mean arterial pressure (MAP) leveled off after 50 to 60 years. These findings were mirrored in the NHANES study and highlighted the age-related pattern of increasing rates of isolated systolic hypertension (ISH) for individuals 50 years or older.[4] In the population younger than 50 years, isolated diastolic hypertension was the most common type of hypertension in untreated individuals (46.9%), whereas ISH became the most prevalent type by the fifth decade (54%), increasing to more than 87% by the sixth decade and after.

Because previous population studies were limited to adults younger than 75 years,[5,6] Lloyd Jones and colleagues[7] examined the Framingham Heart Study elderly population older than 80 years. They pooled data from more than 5000 elderly patients and grouped them according to the Joint National Committee on Detection, Evaluation, and Treatment of High Blood Pressure (JNC) VII stages and ages younger than 60 years, 60 to 79 years, and older than 80 years. As expected, they confirmed the rising prevalence of hypertension with age—27.3%, 63%, and 74% of those younger than 60 years, 60 to 79 years, and older than 80 years, respectively. In addition, the prevalence of stage II hypertension increased with age 20%, 52%, and 60% in men younger than 60 years, 60 to 79 years, and older than 80 years, respectively. Women followed similar trends.

VASCULAR CHANGES WITH AGE

The hemodynamic patterns observed with age can be explained by understanding the composition of arteries, blood pressure components, and age-related vascular changes. Arteries are composed of a balance of elastin and collagen, with the ratio decreasing from central to peripheral arteries in young, normal, and healthy individuals. The elastin is more compliant and provides a cushioning function by expanding during systole and storing some of the stroke volume. During diastole, elastic recoil ignites peripheral runoff of the remainder of the stroke volume.[3,8] With each heartbeat, there is a pulse wave that is emitted that travels down the vascular tree (away from the heart) and is reflected back at bifurcations and the level of small resistance arteries. At any point in time, the pulse wave morphology is represented by the summation of the incident (forward-traveling) and reflected (backward-traveling) pressure waves. Augmentation of the waveform depends on pulse wave velocity (PWV) and impedance—vascular stiffness of the artery. The young have low impedance and PWV, allowing the pulse wave to return during diastole and thereby adding to the DBP.[3,8,9] Patterns of wave summation change with age are discussed later.

The two major physiologic components of blood pressure are MAP, the integrated mean of the pulsatile arterial pressure waveform, and PP, the variation in pressure around the mean. MAP is a function of cardiac output (CO) and systemic vascular resistance (SVR), as indicated in the following equation: MAP = CO × SVR. Both SBP and DBP increase with SVR. Up to 50 years, there is a dominance of SVR on blood pressure and thus MAP in systemic hemodynamics, representing a dual rise in both SBP and DBP. This is because small-vessel resistance is greater than large-vessel resistance. From 50 to 60 years, there is a transition of dominance from MAP to PP as large-vessel stiffness becomes greater than small-vessel resistance.[3,8]

With age, there is an increase in arterial stiffness because of time-dependent fracturing and disarray of elastin replaced by collagen proliferation and calcium deposits called arteriosclerosis.[3,8,10] In central arteries, this leads to a decreased ratio of elastin to collagen and, thus, stiffer arteries. This becomes important when considering the rising SBP and PP and decreasing DBP after 60 years. Stiff arteries have decreased elastic capacity and diminished elastic recoil of the capacitance arteries, causing a quicker runoff of stroke volume and lower central blood volume and pressure at the beginning of diastole. There is also an amplified PWV, causing early return of pulse waves in late systole, rather than diastole. The early return of reflected waves sums on the systolic pressure, and the lack of late returning waves, means less summing on the DBP. Thus, SBP increases, DBP decreases, and PP becomes a surrogate marker for increasing arterial stiffness.[3,9]

EVOLUTION OF JNC GUIDELINES

During the last century, we have gone from recognizing hypertension as a medical problem, to an early focus on DBP, to discovering the importance of SBP as the predominant blood pressure component predictive of CVD.[11] In the 1950s, severe diastolic hypertension was initially the focus of treatment because of the associated increased mortality in the young and the thought that systolic hypertension was part of the natural aging process. In addition, effective treatments for hypertension were limited. The trials responsible for public policy change were the Veterans Affairs (VA) Cooperative trials, in 1967 and 1970, that showed treating DBP 104 to 129 mm Hg protected against stroke and heart failure. This led to the creation of the National High Blood Pressure Education Program and eventually the first Report of the JNC in 1976. Given the positive VA trials in treating DBP, it is obvious why early guidelines set goals based on DBP. However, as early as 1971, Kannel and colleagues[12] with the Framingham Heart Study first reported that SBP had a stronger association with CHD than did DBP. But it was not until after the convincing 1988 Multiple Risk Factor Intervention Trial (MRFIT),[13–15] discussed later, confirmed these findings that SBP was given equal importance in National Guidelines in JNC V (1992).

The most recent US hypertension guidelines—JNC VII,[6] published in 2003—are the current clinical standard for the prevention, detection, evaluation, and treatment of hypertension. The JNC VII report recognizes that SBP elevation confers at least as much risk for adverse events as DBP elevation and recommends that for middle-aged and older hypertensives SBP should be the primary target for staging of blood pressure and initiation of therapy. Moreover, global risk assessment for CVD, that is, consideration of additional risk factors, is recommended in decision making for treatment of hypertension. The current JNC VII classification is shown in **Table 1**. Treatment classification and blood pressure goals are discussed later.

IMPORTANCE OF SBP IN OLDER ADULTS

As indicated by the current JNC guidelines, SBP is recognized as a more robust marker for CVD risk than DBP, especially in the elderly. As previously mentioned,

Table 1
Blood Pressure Staging System of the Seventh Report of the Joint National Committee on Prevention, Detection, Evaluation, and Treatment of High Blood Pressure[6]

JNC VII Blood Pressure Stage	Blood Pressure Range
Normal	SBP <120 *and* DBP <80 mm Hg
Prehypertension	SBP 120–139 *or* DBP 80–89 mm Hg
Stage 1 hypertension	SBP 140–159 *or* DBP 90–99 mm Hg
Stage 2 hypertension	SBP $\geq$ 160 *or* DBP $\geq$ 100 mm Hg

Data from Chobanian AV, Bakris GL, Black HR, et al. Seventh report of the Joint National Committee on Prevention, Detection, Evaluation, and Treatment of High Blood Pressure. Hypertension 2003;42(6):1206–52.

Kannel and colleagues[12] first described the greater predictive value of SBP compared with that of DBP, but it was not generally embraced until MRFIT.[13] This was a randomized, multicenter trial to study the effect of an intervention program on blood pressure, serum cholesterol, and cigarette smoking intervention on mortality and the incidence of CHD. Between 1973 and 1975, more than 300,000 men aged 35 to 57 years were screened for this trial and then followed for mortality outcomes. Men older than 50 years with ISH (SBP > 160, DBP < 90 mm Hg) had the highest 12-year CHD and mortality rates compared with those of diastolic hypertensive and normotensive patients. When all participants were stratified into quintiles of SBP or DBP, risks for each SBP quintile were the same or higher than those for the corresponding quintile of DBP (**Fig. 1**).[14] Similar findings were observed when patients were stratified into deciles of SBP and DBP.[15] Finally, when men were stratified by JNC level of SBP and DBP, SBP was associated with greater risk for CHD mortality than DBP in each JNC blood pressure stage.

Specifically in the older population, SBP has been shown to be a robust predictor of CHF, CHD, and total mortality.[16–19] For example, in the Cardiovascular Health Study of older Americans (**Table 2**), a one standard deviation increment in SBP was associated with higher adjusted risk for CHD and stroke than was a one standard deviation increment in DBP (or PP). In models with SBP and DBP together or SBP and PP together, SBP consistently dominated as the greater risk factor.[19]

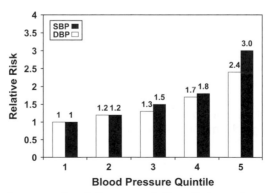

Fig. 1. Relative risk of coronary heart disease mortality with increasing systolic and diastolic blood pressure. (*Data from* Neaton JD, Wentworth D. Serum cholesterol, blood pressure, cigarette smoking, and death from coronary heart disease. Overall findings and differences by age for 316,099 white men. Multiple Risk Factor Intervention Trial Research Group. Arch Intern Med 1992;152(1):56–64.)

Table 2			
Risks for CVD associated with different components of blood pressure in the Cardiovascular Health Study[19]			
		Adjusted Hazards Ratio (95% CI)	
	1 Standard Deviation	Myocardial Infarction	Stroke
Systolic blood pressure	21.4 mm Hg	1.24 (1.15–1.35)	1.34 (1.21–1.47)
Diastolic blood pressure	11.2 mm Hg	1.13 (1.04–1.22)	1.29 (1.17–1.42)
Pulse pressure	18.5 mm Hg	1.21 (1.12–1.31)	1.21 (1.10–1.34)

Data from Psaty BM, Furberg CD, Kuller LH, et al. Association between blood pressure level and the risk of myocardial infarction, stroke, and total mortality: the cardiovascular health study. Arch Intern Med 2001;161(9):1183–92.

In fact, when DBP is considered in the context of the SBP level, an inverse association for DBP and CHD risk has been observed. Franklin and colleagues[20] demonstrated that, at any specified level of SBP, relative risks for CHD *decreased* with increasing DBP. For example, at an SBP of 150 mm Hg, the estimated hazards ratio for CHD was 1.8 if the DBP was 70 mm Hg but only approximately 1.3 if the DBP was 95 mm Hg. The higher the SBP level, the steeper was the decline in CHD risk with increasing DBP. These findings suggest that the predictive value of PP and SBP and DBP diverge. PP is discussed in the next section.

PULSE PRESSURE

In recent literature, PP has been shown to be associated significantly with incident CHD, heart failure, and stroke, especially in older individuals.[9,18-26] There has been significant discussion of whether PP is a better marker of risk than SBP. Recently, a study from the Chicago Heart Association Detection Project in Industry took advantage of a large cohort of more than 30,000 men and women free of CVD and not receiving treatment for hypertension at baseline to examine this issue.[9] This cohort was followed for 33 years and CHD, HF, and stroke outcomes were examined, focusing not just on measures of association (eg, hazards ratios) as in previous studies but also measures of predictive utility. Consistent with some of the prior literature, this large study with extended follow-up showed that PP was a weaker predictor of stroke, CHD, and heart failure outcomes than SBP and other blood pressure measures. There were 11,452 deaths: 745 were attributed to stroke, 2812 to coronary disease, and 599 to heart failure. In univariate analyses, the hazards ratios for stroke death per standard deviation of pulse, systolic, and diastolic pressure, respectively, were 1.49, 1.75, and 1.71. Likelihood ratio chi^2 (134.3, 302.0, and 232.6, respectively), Bayes information criteria values (15,142, 14,974, and 15,044, respectively), and areas under receiver-operating characteristic curves (0.59, 0.64, and 0.63, respectively) all indicated better predictive utility for systolic and diastolic compared with that of PP (**Fig. 2**). These results were representative also of CHD and heart failure in the oldest age group in this study, which included those 60 years or older.

The results highlight the major limitation of PP. Like MAP, PP incorporates information from two blood pressure components (SBP and DBP) and should, therefore, improve classification and risk stratification. However, unlike MAP, PP is "floating;" it has no relation to an absolute blood pressure level. For example, a PP of 60 mm Hg could be associated with blood pressure of 180/120 mm Hg or one of 120/60 mm Hg.

BLOOD PRESSURE GOALS

Given the importance of both SBP and DBP across the age spectrum, both are included in the current JNC VII guidelines (see **Table 2**). However, the new guidelines

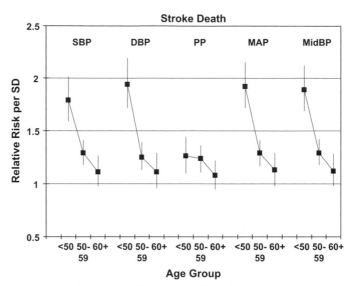

Fig. 2. Relative risk of stroke death with increasing blood pressure by age group. (*Data from* Mosley WJ 2nd, Greenland P, Garside DB, et al. Predictive utility of pulse pressure and other blood pressure measures for cardiovascular outcomes. Hypertension 2007;49(6):1256–64.)

include an emphasis on the robust predictive value of SBP and reclassified the previously "normal" and "high-normal" levels (ie, SBP 120–139 mm Hg or DBP 80–89 mm Hg) to "prehypertension" to place greater emphasis on prevention of hypertension. Individuals are classified into their blood pressure stages on the basis of both SBP and DBP levels. When a disparity exists between SBP and DBP stages, patients are classified into the higher stage.[4] However, the majority of patients are correctly classified by their SBP. Lloyd-Jones and colleagues reported in more than 3500 men and women (mean age, 58 years) that 64.6% of subjects had congruent stages of SBP and DBP, 31.6% were upstaged on the basis of SBP, and 3.8% on the basis of DBP; thus, SBP alone correctly classified JNC VI stage in ~96.6% of the subjects. Among subjects older than 60 years, SBP alone correctly classified 99% of subjects; in those younger than 60 years, SBP alone correctly classified 95%.[7] The JNC blood pressure guidelines have been largely informed by the Prospective Cohorts Study and supported by several other studies.[6,13,17,27] The Prospective study pooled 1 million adults with no previous vascular disease from 61 prospective observational studies to study the age-specific relevance of blood pressure to cause specific mortality. Data from more than 56,000 decedents revealed that risks for CVD death increase in a continuous and graded fashion beginning at levels as low as an SBP of 115 mm Hg and DBP of 75 mm Hg and possibly lower. For each 20-mm Hg increment in SBP or each 10-mm Hg increment in DBP, there was approximately a doubling of risk for stroke death and for ischemic heart disease death in both men and women. This study emphasizes the risk of CVD with rising BP and defines a starting point for risk stratification, which starts in the "normal range." For example, a patient with an SBP of 135 mm Hg has twice the risk of a vascular event than that of a patient with an SBP of 115 mm Hg at any age.

Vasan and colleagues[27] further explored the risk of high blood pressure even in the "high-normal" group as previously classified in JNC VI. Individuals with high-normal blood pressure (SBP 130–139 mm Hg or DBP 85–89 mm Hg, or both) were specifically studied with regard to absolute and relative risk of CVD. These "prehypertensive" levels of BP were associated with significantly elevated multivariable-adjusted relative risk for CVD of 2.5 in women and 1.6 in men, compared with that of optimal blood pressure (SBP <120 mm Hg and DBP <80 mm Hg).

BLOOD PRESSURE TREATMENT IN THE ELDERLY

Despite the known threat of elevated BP and the national initiative for blood pressure control, there is poor adherence to guidelines. In a community-based cohort from the Framingham Heart Study, Lloyd-Jones and colleagues[28] studied more than 5000 men and women to examine the rates of hypertension treatment, control, and cardiovascular risks among persons older than 80 years. The patients were separated into three groups: younger than 60 years, 60 to 79 years, and older than 80 years. As shown in previous studies,[1,2,4] the prevalence of hypertension and drug treatment increased with advancing age; however, blood control was inadequate. In the three groups from young to old, control rates were 38%, 36%, and 38%, respectively, in men (P = .30) and 38%, 28%, and 23%, respectively, in women (P<.001). Among participants aged 80 years or older, major cardiovascular event rates during follow-up of up to 6 years progressively increased with the stage of hypertension—9.5% of the normal group, 19.8% of the pre-hypertension group (hazards ratio [HR], 1.9; 95% confidence interval [CI], 0.9–3.9), 20.3% of the stage 1 hypertension group (HR, 1.8; 95% CI, 0.8–3.7), and 24.7% of the stage 2 or treated hypertension group (HR, 2.4; 95% CI, 1.2–4.6). The observed reluctance to treat the elderly older than 80 years to date may be due to studies showing a benefit from a CVD perspective but an increase in all-cause mortality.[29,30]

There have been several studies showing a benefit of treating hypertension in patients older than 60 years.[31–33] A landmark trial in 1991 from the Systolic Hypertension in the Elderly Program (SHEP)[31] group provided substantial evidence in treating hypertension in the elderly. This was a multicenter, randomized, double-blind, placebo-controlled study that evaluated and followed 4736 men and women older than 60 years for an average of 4.5 years. They were randomized to treatment of ISH (SBP > 160 mm Hg, DBP < 90 mm Hg) with chlorthalidone or atenolol versus placebo. The mean age was 72 years, and 57% were women. The average blood pressure 5 years after randomization was 155/72 mm Hg for the placebo group and 143/68 mm Hg for the active treatment group. This resulted in a significant relative risk reduction for stroke of 36%, for CHD of 27%, and for all cause-mortality of 13%.

A meta-analysis in 2000 (largely from SHEP, The Systolic Hypertension in Europe Trial [Syst-Eur], Systolic Hypertension in China, mannose receptor C type 2), pooled 15,693 patients older than 60 years (mean age, 70 years) with ISH, SBP more than 160 mm Hg, DBP less than 95 mm Hg, analyzing the effect of hypertension treatment on cardiovascular outcomes.[34] Average BP was 174/83 mm Hg, and average decrease in BP with treatment was 5.96% for SBP and 4.9% for DBP. Active treatment significantly reduced total mortality by 13%, CHD death by 18%, and stroke by 26%. Clearly, we can see that treatment of hypertension in the elderly at least up to 70 years is beneficial to overall health and mortality.

Treatment of hypertension in elderly patients older than 80 years was not evaluated specifically in prospective trials until the Hypertension in the Very Elderly Trial (HYVET)[35] study was recently published. Before this study, a meta-analysis by the INDANA[30] group of 1670 individuals 80 years or older from a number of clinical antihypertensive trials (mostly from SHEP and Syst-Eur) evaluated the effects of treatment on CVD and mortality. Events were reduced by 34%, 22% and 39%, respectively, for stroke, total CVD, and heart failure, but there was no cardiovascular mortality benefit. Of potential concern, the analysis suggested a 6% increase in all-cause mortality. The lack of primary data addressing this issue led to the design of the HYVET study.

The HYVET[35] trial was a randomized, prospective trial of 3845 participants older than 80 years, with a mean age of 83 years (range, 80–105 years), with a mean follow-up of 2 years (range, 0–6.5 years). Of those randomized, 61% were women, and 12% had prior CVD, including 7% with prior stroke, 3% with prior MI, and 3% with heart failure. The mean baseline BP was 173/91 mm Hg (32% had ISH). Patients were randomized to a diuretic or placebo. An angiotensin-converting enzyme (ACE) inhibitor was added if necessary to achieve a goal BP of 150/80 mm Hg. Active treatment was associated with a significant 30% relative risk reduction in fatal and nonfatal stroke and 39% reduction in stroke death alone. CVD deaths were reduced by 23%. All-cause mortality was also significantly reduced by 21%. The number needed to treat with active therapy to prevent one death was 40 patients during 2 years. Also notable was the substantially lower rate of heart failure with active treatment (22 vs 57/1000/y; 64% relative risk reduction; $P<.001$).

The HYVET trial answers an important question and makes a profound statement in the treatment of blood pressure in individuals older than 80 years. Physicians can feel comfortable prescribing antihypertensives for their elderly patients and know that there will be a potential mortality benefit. An initial goal of less than 150/less than 80 mm Hg appears to be a safe and reasonably attainable target for most older patients with stage II hypertension and was achieved with ease with one to two antihypertensive medications. A lingering question regarding BP treatment in older individuals is whether there are levels that could be too low that might be associated with increased risk—popularly known as the "J-curve" phenomenon.

J-CURVE PHENOMENON

Past studies have suggested a J-curve phenomenon in treating blood pressure specifically related to DBP, meaning that there is a DBP level that, if surpassed, could be associated with increased risk. It is postulated that a DBP that is too low could decrease coronary perfusion and thus contribute to a poor outcome. There is discussion about whether this is due to a widened PP in patients with ISH, representing central artery impedance, or whether it is irrespective of SBP. In addition, it is thought by some that this may be relevant only in patients with manifest CHD.

The Prospective Collaboration,[17] discussed previously, examined their data for a J-curve effect with declining DBP and found a J-curve that was statistically significant and noted at all ages for ischemic heart disease, stroke, and other vascular mortalities. This study did not account for concurrent SBP.

In 1991, a Framingham study by D'Agostino and colleagues[36] evaluated more than 5000 patients for the J-curve relation and compared those with and without a history of MI. They found a significant J-shaped relation between CHD death and DBP but not SBP. However, this study also did not take into account a concurrent SBP.

A Framingham Study in 2004 by Kannel and colleagues[37] prospectively tested the hypothesis that an increased PP is responsible for the increase in CVD incidence with declining DBP. The study had more than 7000 men and women aged 35 to 80 years. The 10-year risk of 951 nonfatal CVD events and 204 CVD deaths was estimated at diastolic pressures of less than 80 mm Hg, 80 to 90 mm Hg, and more than 90 mm Hg, according to concomitant SBP. As DBP was decreased for fixed SBP, a J-curve relation was seen only when SBP was greater than 140 mm Hg, which persisted with adjustment for age and associated CVD risk factors. This study suggested that PP was responsible for the increased mortality and not low DBP alone.

Contrary to the prior Framingham Study, the smaller Helsinki Ageing Study found a J-curve effect even when accounting for SBP.[38] This study consisted of more than 500 subjects aged 70 to 85 years followed for 5 years. An inverse relationship between SBP and DBP and mortality was shown as well a J-curve relationship with DBP and mortality in those aged 75 years but not in the 80- and 85-year-old group. Although this study found a J-curve relationship, it is contrary to the increasing CVD mortality with rising SBP and DBP seen in the larger prospective studies, mentioned previously.[17,37] Moreover, this study did not report comorbidities that may have been confounders.

In addition to epidemiology studies, blood pressure treatment studies also evaluated for J-curve effect, namely the SHEP,[31] Sys-Eur,[32] and Sys-China[33] groups. The SHEP study randomized more than 4000 patients 60 years or older with ISH (SBP >160 mm Hg and DBP <90 mm Hg) to thiazide, beta blocker, or placebo. This study showed reduction in incidence of hemorrhagic and ischemic stroke with no evidence of harm in treatment of blood pressure less than 90 mm Hg. Staessen and colleagues[32] evaluated more than 4500 patients older than 60 years with 160 to 219 SBP and DBP less than 95 treated with a calcium channel blocker and a possible ace inhibitor and/or thiazide versus placebo. They achieved a significant reduction in stroke mortality and cardiovascular events regardless of DBP. Finally, Wang and colleagues[33] with the Sys-China group evaluated more than 1200 patients who were 60 years or older with a BP of 160 to 219 SBP and DBP less than 95 randomly assigned to treatment of BP with a calcium channel blocker and possible ace inhibitor and/or thiazide versus placebo. They also achieved a reduction of risk of all cardiovascular events including stroke and MI irrespective of the decrease in DBP.

Thus, as seen by multiple epidemiologic trials and treatment trials, the J-curve may largely be related to large PPs as seen when DBP is evaluated with concurrent SBP. In addition, patients with a history of previous MI may be at increased risk for future cardiovascular events with low DBP.

In conclusion, we have shown that there is a clear association between hypertension and CVD and mortality. This is especially relevant as age increases and the burden of hypertension becomes greater. Our poor job in treating hypertension in the elderly was perhaps secondary to reservations regarding the safety of antihypertensive treatment in this population, including those older than 80 years. However, multiple trials, such as SHEP,[31] MRFIT,[13] Sys-Eur,[32] Sys-China,[33] and most recently the HYVET[35] trial, have shown us that not only is it safe to treat hypertension in the elderly but also that it will decrease cardiovascular events and mortality. We should, therefore, be committed to liberally treating hypertension in our patients regardless of their age.

REFERENCES

1. National Center for Health Statistics (U.S.). Health, United States, 2007. With Chartbook on Trends in the Health of Americans. Hyattsville (MD): Public Health Service, Centers for Disease Control and Prevention. Washington, DC: US Department of Health and Human Services; 2007.
2. Levy D, Larson MG, Vasan RS, et al. The progression from hypertension to congestive heart failure. JAMA 1996;275(20):1557–62.
3. Franklin SS, Gustin WT, Wong ND, et al. Hemodynamic patterns of age-related changes in blood pressure. The Framingham Heart Study. Circulation 1997; 96(1):308–15.

4. Franklin SS, Jacobs MJ, Wong ND, et al. Predominance of isolated systolic hypertension among middle-aged and elderly US hypertensives: analysis based on National Health and Nutrition Examination Survey (NHANES) III. Hypertension 2001;37(3):869–74.
5. Burt VL, Cutler JA, Higgins M, et al. Trends in the prevalence, awareness, treatment, and control of hypertension in the adult US population. Data from the health examination surveys, 1960 to 1991. Hypertension 1995;26(1):60–9.
6. Chobanian AV, Bakris GL, Black HR, et al. Seventh report of the Joint National Committee on Prevention, Detection, Evaluation, and Treatment of High Blood Pressure. Hypertension 2003;42(6):1206–52.
7. Lloyd-Jones DM, Evans JC, Larson MG, et al. Differential impact of systolic and diastolic blood pressure level on JNC-VI staging. Joint National Committee on Prevention, Detection, Evaluation, and Treatment of High Blood Pressure. Hypertension 1999;34(3):381–5.
8. Izzo JL, Sica DA, Black HR, et al. Hypertension primer. 4th edition. Philadelphia: Lippincott Williams & Wilkins; 2008.
9. Mosley WJ 2nd, Greenland P, Garside DB, et al. Predictive utility of pulse pressure and other blood pressure measures for cardiovascular outcomes. Hypertension 2007;49(6):1256–64.
10. Izzo JL Jr, Levy D, Black HR. Clinical Advisory Statement. Importance of systolic blood pressure in older Americans. Hypertension 2000;35(5):1021–4.
11. Dustan HP. 50th anniversary historical article. Hypertension. J Am Coll Cardiol 1999;33(3):595–7.
12. Kannel WB, Gordon T, Schwartz MJ. Systolic versus diastolic blood pressure and risk of coronary heart disease. The Framingham study. Am J Cardiol 1971;27(4):335–46.
13. Rutan GH, Kuller LH, Neaton JD, et al. Mortality associated with diastolic hypertension and isolated systolic hypertension among men screened for the Multiple Risk Factor Intervention Trial. Circulation 1988;77(3):504–14.
14. Neaton JD, Wentworth D. Serum cholesterol, blood pressure, cigarette smoking, and death from coronary heart disease. Overall findings and differences by age for 316,099 white men. Multiple Risk Factor Intervention Trial Research Group. Arch Intern Med 1992;152(1):56–64.
15. Neaton JD, Keller L, Stamler J, et al. Impact of systolic and diastolic blood pressure on cardiovascular mortality. 2nd edition. New York: Raven Press; 1995.
16. Franklin SS, Larson MG, Khan SA, et al. Does the relation of blood pressure to coronary heart disease risk change with aging? The Framingham Heart Study. Circulation 2001;103(9):1245–9.
17. Lewington S, Clarke R, Qizilbash N, et al. Age-specific relevance of usual blood pressure to vascular mortality: a meta-analysis of individual data for one million adults in 61 prospective studies. Lancet 2002;360(9349):1903–13.
18. Haider AW, Larson MG, Franklin SS, et al. Systolic blood pressure, diastolic blood pressure, and pulse pressure as predictors of risk for congestive heart failure in the Framingham Heart Study. Ann Intern Med 2003;138(1):10–6.
19. Psaty BM, Furberg CD, Kuller LH, et al. Association between blood pressure level and the risk of myocardial infarction, stroke, and total mortality: the cardiovascular health study. Arch Intern Med 2001;161(9):1183–92.
20. Franklin SS, Khan SA, Wong ND, et al. Is pulse pressure useful in predicting risk for coronary heart Disease? The Framingham heart study. Circulation 1999;100(4):354–60.
21. Chae CU, Pfeffer MA, Glynn RJ, et al. Increased pulse pressure and risk of heart failure in the elderly. JAMA 1999;281(7):634–9.

22. Domanski MJ, Davis BR, Pfeffer MA, et al. Isolated systolic hypertension: prognostic information provided by pulse pressure. Hypertension 1999;34(3):375–80.
23. Kostis JB, Lawrence-Nelson J, Ranjan R, et al. Association of increased pulse pressure with the development of heart failure in SHEP. Systolic Hypertension in the Elderly (SHEP) Cooperative Research Group. Am J Hypertens 2001;14(8 Pt 1):798–803.
24. Mattace-Raso FU, van der Cammen TJ, van Popele NM, et al. Blood pressure components and cardiovascular events in older adults: the Rotterdam study. J Am Geriatr Soc 2004;52(9):1538–42.
25. Vaccarino V, Holford TR, Krumholz HM. Pulse pressure and risk for myocardial infarction and heart failure in the elderly. J Am Coll Cardiol 2000;36(1):130–8.
26. Miura K, Dyer AR, Greenland P, et al. Pulse pressure compared with other blood pressure indexes in the prediction of 25-year cardiovascular and all-cause mortality rates: The Chicago Heart Association Detection Project in Industry Study. Hypertension 2001;38(2):232 7.
27. Vasan RS, Larson MG, Leip EP, et al. Impact of high-normal blood pressure on the risk of cardiovascular disease. N Engl J Med 2001;345(18):1291–7.
28. Lloyd-Jones DM, Evans JC, Levy D. Hypertension in adults across the age spectrum: current outcomes and control in the community. JAMA 2005;294(4):466–72.
29. Amery A, Birkenhager W, Brixko P, et al. Influence of antihypertensive drug treatment on morbidity and mortality in patients over the age of 60 years. European Working Party on High blood pressure in the Elderly (EWPHE) results: sub-group analysis on entry stratification. J Hypertens Suppl 1986;4(6):S642 7.
30. Gueyffier F, Bulpitt C, Boissel JP, et al. Antihypertensive drugs in very old people: a subgroup meta-analysis of randomised controlled trials. INDANA Group. Lancet 1999;353(9155):793–6.
31. Group SCR. Prevention of stroke by antihypertensive drug treatment in older persons with isolated systolic hypertension. Final results of the Systolic Hypertension in the Elderly Program (SHEP). SHEP Cooperative Research Group. JAMA 1991;265(24):3255–64.
32. Staessen JA, Fagard R, Thijs L, et al. Randomised double-blind comparison of placebo and active treatment for older patients with isolated systolic hypertension. The Systolic Hypertension in Europe (Syst-Eur) Trial Investigators. Lancet 1997;350(9080):757–64.
33. Wang JG, Staessen JA, Gong L, et al. Chinese trial on isolated systolic hypertension in the elderly. Systolic Hypertension in China (Syst-China) Collaborative Group. Arch Intern Med 2000;160(2):211–20.
34. Staessen JA, Gasowski J, Wang JG, et al. Risks of untreated and treated isolated systolic hypertension in the elderly: meta-analysis of outcome trials. Lancet 2000; 355(9207):865–72.
35. Beckett NS, Peters R, Fletcher AE, et al. Treatment of hypertension in patients 80 years of age or older. N Engl J Med 2008;358(18):1887–98.
36. D'Agostino RB, Belanger AJ, Kannel WB, et al. Relation of low diastolic blood pressure to coronary heart disease death in presence of myocardial infarction: the Framingham Study. BMJ 1991;303(6799):385–9.
37. Kannel WB, Wilson PW, Nam BH, et al. A likely explanation for the J-curve of blood pressure cardiovascular risk. Am J Cardiol 2004;94(3):380–4.
38. Hakala SM, Tilvis RS, Strandberg TE. Blood pressure and mortality in an older population. A 5-year follow-up of the Helsinki Ageing Study. Eur Heart J 1997; 18(6):1019–23.

Arterial Compliance in the Elderly: Its Effect on Blood Pressure Measurement and Cardiovascular Outcomes

MaryAnn Lim, MD[a], Raymond R. Townsend, MD[a,b],*

KEYWORDS

- Arterial stiffness • Arterial compliance • Elderly
- Pulse wave velocity • Blood pressure
- Cardiovascular outcomes

"Longevity is a vascular question, which has been well expressed in the axiom that man is only as old as his arteries. To a majority of men death comes primarily or secondarily through this portal. The onset of what may be called physiological arterio-sclerosis depends, in the first place, upon the quality of arterial tissue which the individual has inherited, and secondly upon the amount of wear and tear to which he has subjected it."

—*Sir William Osler, 1898*

More than 100 years since William Osler wrote the above statements, his ideas still hold true. The loss of arterial compliance as a result of the aging of human vasculature contributes to the age-dependent rise in isolated systolic hypertension and is an independent predictor of all-cause mortality and cardiovascular (CV) outcomes. In this article, we begin by providing a brief historical perspective of the study of the pulse wave. We then review the physiology of the normal arterial system, the effects of aging on the arterial system, and the different measures of arterial stiffness. Finally, we review the different studies that consider arterial stiffness in the elderly, its impact on hypertension and CV outcome, and current knowledge on how to prevent vascular stiffness.

[a] Renal Electrolyte and Hypertension Division, Department of Medicine, Hospital of the University of Pennsylvania, 1 Founders Building, 3400 Spruce Street, Philadelphia, PA 19104, USA
[b] Hypertension Program, Hospital of the University of Pennsylvania, Philadelphia, PA 19104, USA
* Corresponding author.
E-mail address: townsend@exchange.upenn.edu (R.R. Townsend).

Clin Geriatr Med 25 (2009) 191–205
doi:10.1016/j.cger.2009.01.001
0749-0690/09/$ – see front matter © 2009 Elsevier Inc. All rights reserved.

HISTORICAL PERSPECTIVE

Interest in the human pulse dates back to as far as 1500 BC, when papyri from the ancient Egyptians described the link, albeit vaguely, between the arterial pulse and the function of the heart.[1] The examination of the pulse was an integral part of traditional Chinese, Indian, and Greek medicine.[1] Examination of the pulse then was more of an art than a science, with no way of objectively recording the human pulse, other than the physician's sensing of it.[1]

It was not until 1628, when William Harvey published his classic monograph *An Anatomical Essay on the Movement of the Heart and Blood in Animals*, that the modern era of understanding the CV system began.[2] By proving that the arterial pulse was the result of cardiac systole, Harvey set the scene for physiologic knowledge of the arterial pulse and for its clinical applications.[1]

The nineteenth century proved to be a golden era in the study of the human pulse, as the development of the sphygmograph by Étienne Marey and its refinement during the next few years by Mahomed, Broadbent, and Mackenzie ushered in the birth of sphygmocardiography, or the art of interpreting the shape of the arterial waveform.[3] Mahomed noted important differences in the shape of the waveform with age and was able to differentiate normotensive patients from those with essential and renovascular hypertension.[1,3] It was also in this century that Moens described the link between arterial elasticity and pulse wave velocity (PWV).[4]

After the sphygmomanometer was introduced following the work of Scipione Riva-Rocci (1896) and Nicolai Korotkoff (1905), which enabled blood pressure (BP) to be recorded accurately, quickly, and noninvasively, sphygmography took a backseat in clinical practice. In the twentieth century, the development of easy-to-use mercury manometers by Otto Frank in contrast to the complex calculation required for PWV further overshadowed the use of pulse wave analysis in clinical practice.[1,4]

In the latter half of the twentieth century, investigators noted that even with equivalent BP control some individuals developed CV disease and target organ damage, whereas others did not.[4] These observations prompted considerations that there was likely to be more than just the measured excursion of the pulse (ie, the systolic and diastolic pressures) responsible for such findings. Vascular mechanics, including pulse contour analysis and arterial stiffness, have, in recent years, been demonstrated to play a role in the development of CV disease.[4] Such observations, along with the development of devices that more easily estimate arterial stiffness and reflected wave characteristics, prompted the renewed interest and research in arterial stiffness and its relationship with CV outcomes.

NORMAL ARTERIAL FUNCTION

The arterial system is a branching network of elastic conduits (large arteries) and high-resistance vessels (small arterioles and capillaries). It has two important and interrelated functions: (1) the conduit function, providing sufficient amount of blood to various tissues of the body, and (2) the capacitance function, converting the intermittent, highly pulsatile flow from the left ventricle into a steady arterial blood flow at the level of the small arteries.[5] The capacitance function is performed mainly by the large central arteries that are relatively rich in elastin and collagen and have a low wall-to-lumen ratio.[6] The elastin fibers are responsible for the mechanical strength of the vasculature at low pressures, and the collagen fibers, at higher pressures.[7]

During systole, a bolus of blood is ejected into the aorta, stretching the aortic wall; in the process, most of the systolic pressure is stored as elastic tensile energy within the wall, hence protecting the small arterioles and capillaries from the potential damage of high-pressure flow.[8] Close to the end of systole, when the left ventricle relaxes and can no longer oppose the tension in the aortic wall, blood begins to flow back into the heart until the aortic valve closes commencing diastole.[8] Having nowhere else to go, the blood continues its passage through the systemic circulation (the coronary circulation included), largely propelled by the elastic energy stored during systole and a modest mean arterial pressure gradient favoring forward flow.[8] Thus, the cushioning function, which stores energy in the elastic walls of compliant vessels such as the aorta, protects small arterioles from high-pressure damage and ensures continuous blood flow and oxygenation to target organs.[5,6] It also minimizes cardiac work, by conserving energy and making the cardiac cycle as efficient as possible.[5,6]

As blood flows out from the heart as a result of left ventricular systole, a propagation wave is generated, which accompanies the flow of blood from the heart to the periphery. This propagation wave is a composite of left ventricular ejection, properties of the blood (such as viscosity), and characteristics of the arterial tree.[4,8] On arrival at branch points or sites of impedance mismatch, this pressure wave is reflected and returned to the heart.[4] The final pressure wave, as seen by an invasive catheter, for example, is the sum of the forward and reflected waves. For maximal efficiency, wave reflection should not add to the pressure generated during systole.[5] The reflected wave should ideally reach the heart during diastole, to sustain the diastolic BP and augment coronary perfusion during diastole.[4,5] **Fig. 1** illustrates this concept.

AGING AND VASCULAR AGING

Aging has been associated with changes in the arterial system at different structural and functional levels. At the macroscopic level, an increase in lumen size[9] as well as an increase in arterial wall thickening, mainly in the intima,[10,11] are observed. At the molecular level, changes from aging consist of the following: (1) increased collagen content and cross-linking, (2) increased elastin fragmentation, and (3) decreased

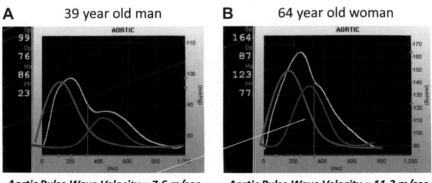

A   39 year old man

Aortic Pulse Wave Velocity = 7.6 m/sec

B   64 year old woman

Aortic Pulse Wave Velocity = 11.3 m/sec

Fig. 1. Aortic waveforms derived from radial artery-based tonometry. The yellow line represents summation waveforms of an outward traveling (*green line*) and backward traveling (*red line*). (A) An aortic waveform from a 39-year-old man with normal BP and a normal aortic PWV of 7.6 m/s. The backward traveling waveform arrives at the end of systole and contributes to the small rise in pressure at the incisura (*green vertical line*) when the aortic valve closes. This mostly diastolic pressure contribution aids in coronary perfusion. (B) A 64-year-old woman with an elevated aortic PWV of 11.3 m/s has a backward traveling wave that arrives earlier in systole contributing to additional systolic pressure. Note, too, the greater amplitude of the backward traveling wave on the right-hand side.

elastin content.[12] Aside from these structural changes, functional changes are also observed in the form of age-associated deterioration in endothelial function.[13,14] All of the above changes contribute to the observed increase in arterial stiffness that accompanies aging.

Arterial stiffness has a marked and progressive effect on the capacitance function. With arterial stiffness, the velocity of both the propagation wave and the reflected wave increases, resulting in an earlier arrival of the reflected wave back to the heart, encroaching upon systole.[4,6,15] This causes an increase in systolic pressure and a decrease in diastolic pressure (leading to a widened pulse pressure). The end result is a higher workload for the heart, decreased coronary perfusion during diastole, and higher pressures that are transmitted to the end organs, such as the kidneys and the brain.[4,6,15]

Increasing arterial stiffness also affects the conduit function. It does this by increasing blood flow during systole when shearing forces are higher.

PROXIMAL AND DISTAL ARTERIAL STIFFNESS

In a healthy arterial bed, the elastic properties of arteries are normally variable—with proximal arteries usually more elastic and distal arteries stiffer.[16] Differences in the molecular, cellular, and histological structures of the arterial wall in different segments of the arterial tree account for this noted heterogeneity.[16,17] Such heterogeneity on the vessel wall has important physiological and pathophysiological consequences.

Imagine a pressure wave propagated along an elastic tube without reflection sites. Eventually, this pressure wave will diminish in size and disappear. Imagine this same pressure wave propagated along an elastic tube with numerous branch points, each of these branch points serving as reflection sites. The pressure wave will get progressively amplified as it moves from central arteries to distal arterioles; the amplification would be even higher if the distal arteries are stiffer, because this would lead to a faster velocity of both propagated wave and reflected wave. This is known as the "amplification phenomenon," and it accounts for the higher amplitude of pressure wave in the peripheral arteries than that in the central arteries.[16]

This amplification phenomenon is less pronounced in the elderly.[5] In fact, when comparing arterial pressures between a 20-year-old and an 80-year-old, if we only look at their brachial systolic BPs (SBPs), only a 20% increase from 120 to 140 mm Hg is evident. However, looking more closely at their aortic pulse pressure, they typically change from 22 to 65 mm Hg, which is actually close to a 200% increase.[5,18]

This shifting trend in using central pressure rather than peripheral brachial pressures to assess CV risk is not limited to the elderly population. In a population of more than 10,000 individuals aged 18 to 92 years, McEniery and colleagues recently showed that more than 70% of individuals with high normal brachial pressure had similar aortic pressures as those in individuals with stage 1 hypertension.[19] Thus, using only brachial BP would miss the overlap of central aortic systolic pressures between those with brachial SBP < 140 and those with SBP $\geq$ 140.[19]

Partly because of the reliance on brachial sphygmomanometer and cuff SBPs, the effects of aging on arterial function have been largely underestimated in the past.[5] Hence, it is imperative that studies on vascular aging not only consider direct measures of vascular compliance and stiffness but also focus on central artery measurements as much as possible.

PULSE WAVE VELOCITY AND OTHER MEASURES OF VASCULAR COMPLIANCE

In the last 20 years, research on arterial stiffness, its measurement, and how it affects CV outcomes has expanded greatly. The assessment of arterial stiffness and complianc can be grouped into three broad categories: (1) measurement of PWV, (2) measurement of arterial distensibility, and (3) assessment of peripheral arterial pressure waveforms.[4]

Measurement of PWV

PWV is defined as the speed of travel of the pressure pulse wave along a specified distance on the vascular bed and can be obtained from any vascular bed accessible to palpation.[3,4,6,20,21] From a mathematical standpoint, PWV is defined using a formula called the Moens-Korteweg equation:

$$PWV = \sqrt{\left(\frac{E_h}{2_{pR}}\right)}$$

where E is the Young's modulus of elasticity of wall material, h is the wall thickness, p is the density of blood and, R is the inside radius of vessel.[20] From this equation, it is evident that PWV is influenced by arterial compliance (which is in turn dependent on elasticity and wall thickness), blood density, and vessel radius. Simplistically stated, the stiffer the artery, the faster the PWV.

The technique of PWV measurement has been validated as simple to learn and reproducible.[22–24] To measure PWV, pulse wave signals are recorded with pressure tonometers positioned over two arterial sites, such as the carotid and femoral arteries. Distances between the two sampling sites are measured (D). In order to determine the time elapsed (Δt) as the wave travels from the more proximal to the more distal site,

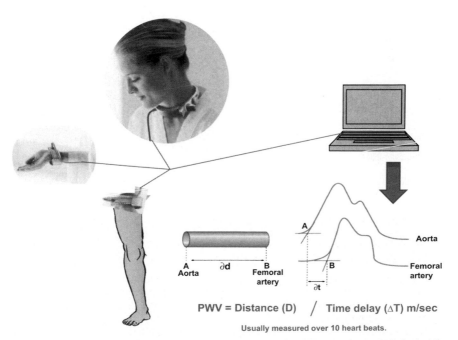

PWV = Distance (D) / Time delay (ΔT) m/sec

Usually measured over 10 heart beats.

Fig. 2. Graphic of woman with neck and wrist segments of a PWV measurement device that records pulsations simultaneously at multiple sites (neck, wrist, thigh, etc). PWV is determined by dividing the distance between measurement sites by the time elapsed between the waveforms sensed at each site.

either two tonometers record the same pulse wave in series (such as the Complior) or a single tonometer records the time elapsed as the pulse wave travels to each site sequentially (such as the SphygmaCor). In the latter case, a timing reference, such as the tip of the QRS complex on the electrocardiogram, is used as a central starting point. PWV is then calculated as follows:

$$PWV = D/\Delta t$$

where D is the distance in meters, and Δt is the time interval in seconds. **Figs. 2** and **3.** illustrates this concept.

A number of limitations in this method should be emphasized.[16] (1) Since PWV is largely influenced by the distance measured, small inaccuracies in measurement of distance, such as those in patients with abdominal obesity, would affect the absolute value of PWV. (2) The pressure wave may be attenuated and delayed in the presence of aortic, iliac, or proximal femoral artery stenosis, thus affecting the measured PWV. (3) The femoral pressure waveform may be technically difficult to obtain in certain patients (ie, obese patients or patients with peripheral artery diseases).

Measurement of Arterial Distensibility

Arterial distensibility is defined as the change in arterial diameter during systole relative to diastole.[20] Decreased distensibility suggests arterial stiffening.

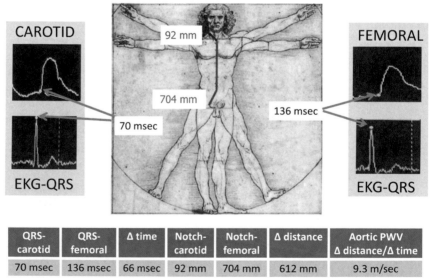

QRS-carotid	QRS-femoral	Δ time	Notch-carotid	Notch-femoral	Δ distance	Aortic PWV Δ distance/Δ time
70 msec	136 msec	66 msec	92 mm	704 mm	612 mm	9.3 m/sec

Fig. 3. Here PWV is measured by recordings made of waveforms (in sequence, instead of simultaneously as in **Fig. 2**) at two different sites of known distance. Since they are not simultaneous, to determine timing lapse at the sites, the tip of the QRS from a surface electrocardiogram is used (typically limb lead II) by averaging waveform times during 10 s of cardiac activity. Once distance is measured and average timing lapse is determined, the PWV is again calculated as distance divided by the delta (difference) in time between the points. In the example shown, it took an average of 70 msec for the waveform foot to be detected at the carotid site and an average of 136 msec for the waveform foot to be detected at the femoral site. The time elapsed is 66 msec.

Ultrasound and a simultaneously recorded BP have been used to measure distensibility and compliance using the following formulas:

Distensibility = $\Delta V / \Delta P \cdot V$

Compliance = $\Delta V / \Delta P$

where ΔV is the change in volume, ΔP is the change in pressure, and V is the volume of the vessel.[3]

The use of this technique is limited to the larger and more accessible arteries and has mainly been used on the brachial, femoral, and carotid arteries and the abdominal aorta. Several images of the vessel wall are obtained per cardiac cycle; a computerized software and wall tracking are then used to compute the maximum and minimum wall areas and volume. Problems with this technique include the following: (1) limited resolution making small changes in vessel wall diameter difficult, (2) operator dependence, (3) concerns about reproducibility and (4) expense of equipment.[3] Aside from these, the BP is usually obtained from a different site (brachial or finger) than the site being imaged by ultrasound, casting further doubts on the reliability of the distensibility and/or compliance measurements.[3] Moreover, inherent differences in muscular arteries such as the brachial artery compared with more elastic arteries such as the aorta, which has a lower wall-to-lumen ratio, further make ultrasound as a measure of arterial stiffness unreliable. Because of all these limitations, the use of ultrasound to measure arterial distensibility has largely been limited to research settings.[3]

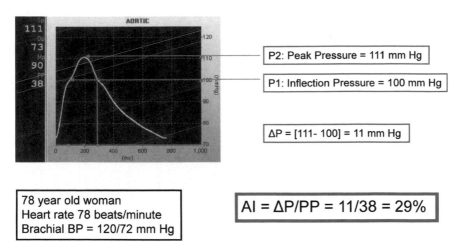

Fig. 4. Aortic waveform derived from applanation tonometry from a 78-year-old woman. Her brachial BP of 120/72 mm Hg was entered into the computer program to calibrate the radial artery waveform. After recording 10 sec of radial artery waveforms of good quality, the software algorithm determined the central aortic pressure profile. In the aortic waveform provided, there is an inflection (first green dot on X-axis) at approximately 100 mm Hg (by the right-hand Y-axis calibration), which is labeled P1. The aortic pressure profile peaks at a value of 111 mm Hg (P2) delineated by the upper green line. The total excursion (or pulse pressure) of the aortic profile is 38 mm Hg (as noted by the lower value in the column of values to the left of the aortic waveform graphic; these values are the central aortic systolic, diastolic, mean, and pulse pressures (PP), reading top to bottom). The PP divided into the value of ?P (which is derived as the delta of peak systolic pressure P2 minus the P1 value; 11 mm Hg) is the Augmentation Index (AI).

Table 1
Epidemiologic studies on aortic stiffness using aortic pulse wave velocity

First Author	Year	Country	Outcome Measures (No. of Events)	Length of Follow-up (y)	Study Population (No.)	Mean Age at Entry(y)	PWV	Hazard Ratio	95% CI	P Value
Blacher et al[30]	1999	France	All-cause mortality (73)	6.0	ESRD (241)	51	1 m/s increase	1.39	1.19–1.62	n/a
—	—	—	All-cause mortality (73)	—	—	—	PWV > 12.0 vs < 9.4 m/s	5.4	2.4–11.9	0.0004
—	—	—	CV mortality (48)	—	—	—	PWV > 12.0 vs < 9.4 m/s	5.9	2.3–15.5	0.002
Guerin et al[36]	2001	France	All-cause mortality (59)	4.3	ESRD	—	Absence of PWV decrease	2.59	1.51–4.43	<0.001
—	—	—	CV mortality (40)	—	—	—	Absence of PWV decrease	2.35	1.23–4.51	0.01
Laurent et al[33]	2001	France	All-cause mortality (107)	9.3	HTN (1980)	50	5 m/s increase	1.34	1.04–1.74	0.02
—	—	—	CV mortality (46)	—	—	—	5 m/s increase	1.51	1.08–2.11	0.03
Meaume et al[37]	2001	France	CV mortality (27)	2.5	Elderly (141)	87	1 m/s increase	1.19	1.03–1.37	0.016
Shoji et al[35]	2001	Japan	All-cause mortality (81)	5.2	ESRD (265)	55	1 m/s increase	1.15	1.03–1.29	<0.05
—	—	—	CV mortality (36)	—	—	—	1 m/s increase	1.18	1.01–1.39	<0.05
Boutouyrie et al[31]	2002	France	CHD events (53)	5.7	HTN (1045)	51	3.5 m/s increase	1.34	1.01–1.79	0.039

Study	Year	Country	Outcome (n)	Follow-up	Population (n)	Age	Measure	HR/RR	95% CI	p
Cruickshank et al[34]	2002	UK	All-cause mortality (219)	10.7	Impaired glucose tolerance (571)	51	1 m/s increase	1.08	1.03–1.14	0.001
Laurent et al[32]	2003	France	Fatal strokes	7.9	HTN (1715)	51	4 m/s increase	1.72	1.48–1.96	<0.001
Sutton-Tyrell et al[38]	2005	USA	All-cause mortality (265)	4.6	Elderly (2488)	74	1 log (PWV) unit	1.6	1.2–2.2	<0.05
—	—	—	CV mortality (111)				1 log (PWV) unit	1.80	1.10–2.80	<0.05
Shokawa et al[40]	2005	Japan	CV mortality (14)	10	General population (492)	64	1 m/s increase	1.35	1.12–1.57	<0.01
—	—	—	CV mortality (14)	—	—	—	> 9.9 m/s vs < 9.9 m/s	4.24	1.39–12.96	<0.01
Willum-Hansen et al[41]	2006	Denmark	CV mortality (62)	9.4	General population (1678)	55	3.4 m/s increase	1.2	1.01–1.41	<0.05
Mattace-Raso et al[39]	2006	Netherlands	CHD (101)	4.1	Elderly (2835)	72	Lowest to highest tertiles	2.45	1.29–4.66	0.02
—	—	—	Stroke (63)	—	—	—	Lowest to highest tertiles	2.28	1.05–4.96	0.03

Abbreviations: CI, confidence interval; CHD, coronary heart disease; ESRD, end-stage renal disease; HTN, hypertension; m/s, meters/second; n/a, not available.

Assessment of Peripheral Arterial Pressure Waveforms

As described earlier, the arterial pressure waveform is a composite of the forward propagation wave and reflected wave. In a healthy arterial tree, the reflected wave arrives back at the aortic root during diastole. Stiffer arteries generate higher PWVs, resulting in the reflected wave reaching the aortic root at the end of systole and augmenting the late systolic pressure (see **Fig. 1**, panel B). This results in a second systolic peak on the pressure waveform, also known as the inflection point. To estimate the effect of this reflected wave on the pulse pressure, a value called an augmentation index (AI) can be generated in the following fashion:

$$\text{Augmentation index}(AI) = (P2 - P1)/pp$$

where $P2$ and $P1$ are the peak systolic peak pressure and inflection pressure, respectively, and pp is the pulse pressure.[3,6,16,20] A graphical depiction of the AI is shown in **Fig. 4**. The AI estimates vascular compliance, in that the stiffer the artery, the higher the AI.[3,6,16] AI can be obtained by application of the transfer function to the pressure pulse obtained at the radial or carotid arteries by applanation tonometry.[6,16]

First, in considering AI as a surrogate marker of arterial stiffness, it is important to recognize that in contrast to aortic PWV, which is the speed of wave travel and is thus a direct measure of arterial stiffness, AI is an *indirect* measure of arterial stiffness, as it is dependent on other factors aside from PWV.[16] These include the amplitude of the reflected wave, the distance to the reflectance point (s), and the duration and pattern of ventricular ejection.[16] Second, certain pathophysiologic conditions and drugs may change central pulse pressure and AI without necessarily changing PWV.[16,25,26] Third, AI has been shown to be more sensitive to heart rate and height than PWV.[16] Fourth, gender has been found to influence AI in that women have a higher AI than that of men.[27] Finally, in the elderly population, aortic PWV was found to be a better measure of arterial stiffness than AI in at least 2 studies.[28,29] Indeed, the position statement put forth by the European expert consensus on arterial stiffness is to not use AI and PWV interchangeably but to use AI coupled with PWV to determine the contribution of aortic stiffness to wave reflections.[16]

ARTERIAL STIFFNESS AND CARDIOVASCULAR OUTCOMES

The largest amount of epidemiologic data with regard to arterial stiffness and its relationship to CV outcomes is that obtained via aortic PWV (carotid-femoral PWV). The first direct evidence that increased aortic stiffness is a strong and independent predictor of CV mortality was shown in a cohort of 241 hemodialysis patients followed prospectively by Blacher and colleagues in 1999.[30] Subsequently, aortic stiffness has been shown to be an independent predictor of all-cause and CV mortalities, fatal and nonfatal coronary events, and fatal strokes in patients with uncomplicated essential hypertension,[31–33] type 2 diabetes,[34] end-stage renal disease (ESRD),[35,36] elderly subjects,[37–39] and the general population[40,41] independent of other CV risk factors. The pertinent details of these studies are summarized in **Table 1**.

Worth special mention is a prospective study by Guerin and colleagues of 150 dialysis patients with hypertension.[36] The patients' BPs were lowered by targeting their dry weight; they were then randomly assigned to either an angiotensin-converting enzyme inhibitor ACE-I or a calcium channel blocker. Of the 150 patients, 59 died during the 4-year follow-up. The important observation that was made was that the aortic PWV of those who died during follow-up began at a higher average value and did not decline even with documented reduction in brachial BPs.

One possible explanation for this is the fact that aortic stiffness integrates the damage of CV risk factors on the arterial wall during a long period of time, whereas BP, glycemia, and lipids fluctuate over time, and their values, recorded at the time of risk assessment, may not reflect the true values damaging the arterial wall.[4,16] Thus, lowering BP and lipid values and improving glycemia control in a few weeks may improve CV risk scores, but without attenuating arterial stiffness, which may take a longer period of time, or may be partially irreversible, an improvement in CV mortality may not actually be seen.[16]

MODIFYING ARTERIAL STIFFNESS

A number of small studies have reported improvement in arterial compliance with several pharmacologic and nonpharmacologic interventions.

Dietary and lifestyle changes that have been shown to reduce arterial stiffness include the following: low-salt diet,[42,43] moderate alcohol consumption,[44] garlic powder,[45] alpha-linoleic acid,[46] fish oil,[47] dietary isoflavins,[48] and weight loss.[49] Surprisingly, contradictory results have been found with aerobic exercise and arterial stiffness.[49–51] Hormone replacement therapy has also been shown to have a positive effect on arterial stiffness.[52,53]

Pharmacologic treatments that are able to reduce arterial stiffness include the following: antihypertensive medications (such as diuretics, ACE-I, angiotensin receptor blockers, beta blockers, and calcium channel blockers),[54–61] medications for treatment of congestive heart failure (ACE-I, nitrate, and aldosterone antagonists),[62,63] lipid-lowering agents,[64] thiazolidinediones,[65] sildenafil,[66] and advanced glycation end-product breakers such as alagebrium.[67]

SUMMARY

Aging is associated with a number of structural and functional changes that are thought to contribute to arterial stiffness. Increasing arterial stiffness has been associated with increasing central SBP and has been shown to be an independent predictor of all-cause mortality and CV outcomes. Sphygmomanometric measurements of brachial SBP do not fully reflect central aortic pressure profiles and may thus be falsely reassuring. Measurement of aortic PWV is the best available noninvasive measure of aortic stiffness and correlates well with CV outcomes.

Numerous studies with pharmacologic and nonpharmacologic interventions have shown improvement of aortic PWV values. In spite of these studies, several questions remain unanswered: (1) Will improvement in arterial stiffness translate into improved CV morbidity and mortality? and (2) Will normalizing arterial stiffness be more effective at improving CV outcomes than the present standard of care? The study by Guerin and colleagues[36] may have partially addressed the first question (at least in ESRD patients), but further studies need to be done to completely settle these issues.

REFERENCES

1. Vlachopolous C, R'Oourke M. Genesis of the normal and abnormal arterial pulse. Curr Probl Cardiol 2000;25:303–67.
2. Harvey W. Anatomical essay on the movement of the heart and blood in animals. translator. In: Harvey W, Franklin KJ, editors. The circulation of the blood and other writings. London: Everyman's Library; 1963.

3. Mackenzie IS, Wilkinson IB, Cockroft JR. Assessment of arterial stiffness in clinical practice. Q J Med 2002;95:67–74.
4. DeLoach SS, Townsend RR. Vascular stiffness: its measurement and significance for epidemiologic and outcome studies. Clin J Am Soc Nephrol 2008;3: 184–92.
5. O'Rouke MF. Arterial aging: pathophysiological principles. Vasc Med 2007;12: 329–41.
6. Jani B, Rajkumar C. Ageing and vascular aging. Postgrad Med J 2006;82: 357–62.
7. Bank AJ, Wong H, Holte JE, et al. Contribution of collagen, elastin and smooth muscle to in vivo human brachial artery wall stress and elastic modules. Circulation 1994;12:3263–70.
8. Greenwald SE. Ageing of the conduit arteries. J Pathol 2007;211:157–72.
9. Gesternblith G, Frederiksen J, Yin FC, et al. Echocardiographic assessment of the normal aging population. Circulation 1977;56:273–8.
10. Virmani R, Avolio AP, Mergner WJ, et al. Effect of aging on aortic morphology in populations with high and low prevalence of hypertension and atherosclerosis. Comparison between occidental and Chinese communities. Am J Pathol 1991; 139:1119–29.
11. Nagai Y, Metter EJ, Earley CJ, et al. Increased carotid artery intimal-medial thickness in asymptomatic older subjects with exercise-induced myocardial ischemia. Circulation 1998;98:1504–9.
12. Najjar SS, Lakatta EG. Vascular aging. from molecular to clinical cardiology. In: Runge MS, Patterson C, editors. Contemporary cardiology: principles of molecular cardiology. Totowa (NJ): Human Press Inc; 2005. p. 515–47.
13. Celermajer DS, Sorensen KE, Spiegelhalter DJ, et al. Aging is associated with endothelial dysfunction in healthy men years before the age-related decline in women. J Am Coll Cardiol 1994;24:471–6.
14. Gerhard M, Roddy MA, Creager SJ, et al. Aging progressively impairs endothelial-dependent vasodilation in forearm resistance vessels of humans. Hypertension 1996;27:849–53.
15. Mitchell GF, Parise H, Benjamin EJ, et al. Changes in arterial stiffness and wave reflection with advancing age in healthy men and women: the Framingham heart study. Hypertension 2004;43:1239–45.
16. Laurent S, Cockroft J, Van Bortel L, et al. Expert consensus document on arterial stiffness: methodological issues and clinical applications. Eur Heart J 2006;27: 2588–605.
17. Laurent S, Boutouyrie P, Lacolley P. Structural and genetic bases of arterial stiffness. Hypertension 1994;23:878–83.
18. O'Rourke MF, Hashimoto J. Mechanical factors in arterial aging: a clinical perspective. J Am Coll Cardiol 2007;50:1–13.
19. McEniery CM, Yasmin, McDonell B, et al. Central pressure: variability and impact of cardiovascular risk factors: the Anglo-Cardiff collaborative trail II (ACCT). Hypertension 2008;51:1476–82.
20. Zoungas S, Asmar R. Arterial stiffness and cardiovascular outcome. Clin Exp Pharmacol Physiol 2007;43:647–51.
21. Bramwell JC, Hill AV. The velocity of pulse wave in man. Proc R Soc Lond B Biol Sci 1922;93:298–306.
22. Chen CH, Nevo E, Fetics B, et al. Estimation of central aortic pressure waveform by mathematical transformation of radial tonometry pressure: validation of generalized transfer function. Circulation 1997;95:1827–36.

23. Wilkinson IB, Fuchs SA, Jansen IM, et al. Reproducibility of pulse wave velocity and augmentation index measured by pulse wave analysis. J Hypertens 1999; 16:2079–84.

24. Wimmer NJ, Townsend RR, Joffe MM, et al. Correlation between pulse wave velocity and other measures of arterial stiffness in chronic kidney disease. Clin Nephrol 2007;68(3):133–43.

25. Lemogoum D, Flores G, Van den Abeele W, et al. Validity of pulse pressure and augmentation index as surrogate measures of arterial stiffness during beta-adrenergic stimulation. J Hypertens 2004;22:511–7.

26. Wilkinson IB, MacCallum H, Hupperetz PC, et al. Changes in the derived central pressure waveform and pulse pressure in response to angiotensin II and noradrenaline in man. J Physiol 2001;530:541–50.

27. Hayward CS, Kelly RP. Gender-related differences in the central arterial pressure waveforms. J Am Coll Cardiol 1997;30:1863–71.

28. McEniery CM, Yasmin, Hall IR, et al. Normal vascular aging: differential effects of wave reflection and aortic pulse wave velocity: the Anglo-Cardiff collaborative trial (ACCT). J Am Coll Cardiol 2005;46:1753–60.

29. Vyas M, Izzo JI, Lacourciere Y, et al. Augmentation index and central aortic stiffness in middle-aged to elderly individuals. Am J Hypertens 2007;20:642–7.

30. Blacher J, Guerin AP, Pannier P, et al. Impact of aortic stiffness on survival in end-stage renal disease. Circulation 1999;99:2434–9.

31. Boutouyrie P, Tropeano AI, Asmar R, et al. Aortic stiffness is an independent predictor of primary coronary events in hypertensive patients: a longitudinal study. Hypertension 2002;39:10–5.

32. Laurent S, Katsahian S, Fassot C, et al. Aortic stiffness is an independent predictor of fatal stroke in essential hypertension. Stroke 2003;34:1203–6.

33. Laurent S, Boutouyrie P, Asmar R, et al. Aortic stiffness is an independent predictor of all-cause and cardiovascular mortality in hypertensive patients. Hypertension 2001;37:1236–41.

34. Cruickshank K, RisteL, Anderson SG, et al. Aortic pulse wave velocity and its relationship to mortality in diabetes and glucose intolerance: an integrated index of cardiovascular function? Circulation 2002;106:2085–90.

35. Shoji T, Emoto M, Shinohara K, et al. Diabetes mellitus, aortic stiffness and cardiovascular mortality in end-stage renal disease. J Am Soc Nephrol 2001;12:2117–24.

36. Guerin AP, Blacher J, Pannier B, et al. Impact of aortic stiffness attenuation on survival of patients with end-stage renal failure. Circulation 2001;103:987–92.

37. Meaume S, Benetos A, Henry OF, et al. Aortic pulse wave velocity predicts cardiovascular mortality in subjects > 70 years of age. Arterioscler Thromb Vasc Biol 2001;21:2046–50.

38. Sutton-Tyrell K, Najjar SS, Boudreau RM, et al. Elevated aortic pulse wave velocity, a marker of arterial stiffness, predicts cardiovascular events in well functioning older adults. Circulation 205;111:3384–90.

39. Mattace-Raso FUS, van der Cammen TJM, Hofman A, et al. Arterial stiffness and the risk of coronary heart disease and stroke. The Rotterdam Study. Circulation 2006;113:657–63.

40. Shokawa T, Imazu M, Yamamoto H, et al. Pulse wave velocity predicts cardiovascular mortality: findings from the Hawaii-Los Angeles-Hiroshima study. Circ J 205;69:259–64.

41. Willum-Hansen T, Staessen JA, Torp-Pedersen C. Prognostic value of aortic pulse wave velocity as an index of arterial stiffness in the general population. Circulation 2006;113:664–70.

42. Avolio AP, Clyde KM, beard TC, et al. Improved arterial distensibility in normotensive subjects on a low salt diet. Arteriosclerosis 1986;6:166–9.
43. Gates PE, Tanana H, Hiatt WR, et al. Dietary sodium restriction rapidly improves large elastic artery compliance in older adults with systolic hypertension. Hypertension 2004;44:35–41.
44. Sierkman A, Lebrun CE, van der Schouw YT, et al. Alcohol consumption in relation to aortic stiffness and aortic pulse wave reflections: a cross-sectional study in healthy post-menopausal women. Arterioscler Thromb Vasc Biol 2004;24:342–8.
45. Breithaupt-Grogler K, Ling M, Boudoulas H, et al. Protective effects of chronic garlic intake on elastic properties of aorta in the elderly. Circulation 1997;96:2649–55.
46. Nestel PJ, Pomeroy SE, Sasahara T, et al. Arterial compliance in obese subjects is improved with dietary plan-3 fatty acid from flaxseed oil despite increased LDL oxidizability. Arterioscler Thromb Vasc Biol 1997;17:1163–70.
47. McVeigh GE, Brennan GM, Cohn JN, et al. Fish oil improves arterial compliance in non-insulin dependent diabetes mellitus. Arterioscler Thromb 1994;14:1425–9.
48. van der Schovw YT, Pijpe A, Lebrun CE, et al. Higher usual dietary intake of phytoestrogens is associated with lower aortic stiffness in postmenopausal women. Arterioscler Thromb Vasc Biol 2002;22:1316–22.
49. Balkestein EJ, Van Aggel-Leijssen DP, Van Baak MA, et al. The effects of weight loss with or without exercise training on large artery compliance in healthy obese men. J Hypertens 1999;17:1831–5.
50. Kingwell BA, Berry KL, Cameron JD, et al. Arterial compliance increases after moderate-intensity cycling. Am J Phys 1997;273:H2186–91.
51. Ferrier KE, Waddell TK, Gatzka CD, et al. Aerobic exercise training does not modify large artery compliance in isolated systolic hypertension. Hypertension 2001;38:222–6.
52. Rajkumar C, Kingwell BA, Cameron JD, et al. Hormonal therapy increases arterial compliance in postmenopausal women. J Am Coll Cardiol 1997;30:350–6.
53. Waddell TK, Rajkumar C, Cameron J, et al. Withdrawal of hormonal therapy for 4 weeks decreases arterial compliance in postmenopausal women. J Hypertens 1999;17:413–8.
54. Girerd X, Giannattasio C, Moulin C, et al. Regression of radial artery wall hypertrophy and improvement of carotid artery compliance after long term antihypertensive treatment: the Pericles study. J Am Coll Cardiol 1998;31:1064–73.
55. Asmar RG, Pannier B, Santoni JPh, et al. Reversion of cardiac hypertrophy and reduced arterial compliance after angiotensin converting enzyme inhibition in essential hypertension. Circulation 1988;78:941–50.
56. Kool MJ, Lustermans FA, Breed JG, et al. The influence of perindopril and the diuretic combination amiloride + hydrochlorothiazide on the vessel wall properties of large arteries in hypertensive patients. J Hypertens 1995;13:839–48.
57. Ting CT, Chen CH, Chang MS, et al. Short and long-term effects of antihypertensive drugs on arterial reflections, compliance and impedance. Hypertension 1995;26:524–30.
58. Mahmud A, Feely J. Reduction in arterial stiffness with angiotensin II antagonist is comparable with and additive to ACE inhibition. Am J Hypertens 2002;15:321–5.
59. Karalliedde J, Smith A, DeAngelis L, et al. Valsartan improves arterial stiffness in type 2 diabetes independently of blood pressure lowering. Hypertension 2008;51:1617–23.

60. Topochian J, Asmar R, Sayegh F, et al. Changes in arterial structure and function under trandolapril-verapamil combination in hypertension. Stroke 1999;30: 1056–64.
61. Simon AC, Levenson J, Bouthier JD, et al. Effects of chronic administration of enalapril and propranolol on the large arteries in essential hypertension. J Cardiovasc Pharmacol 1985;7:856–61.
62. Laurent S, Arcaro G, Benestos A, et al. Mechanism of nitrate-induced improvement on arterial compliance depends on vascular territory. J Cardiovasc Pharmacol 1992;19:641–9.
63. White WB, Duprez D, St Hillaire R, et al. Effects of selective aldosterone blocker eplerenone versus the calcium antagonist amlodipine in systolic hypertension. Hypertension 2003;42:1021–6.
64. Ferrier KE, Muhlmann MH, Bagnet JP, et al. Intensive cholesterol reduction lowers blood pressure and improves large artery stiffness in isolated systolic hypertension. J Am Coll Cardiol 2002;9:1020–5.
65. Nakamura T, Matsuda T, Kawagoe Y, et al. Effect of pioglitazone on carotid intima-media thickness and arterial stiffness in type 2 diabetic nephropathy patients. Meta 2004;53:1382–6.
66. Vlachopoulos C, Hirta K, O'Rourke MF. Effect of sildenafil on arterial stiffness and wave reflection. Vasc Med 2003;8:243–8.
67. Kass DA, Shapiro EP, Kawaguchi M, et al. Improved arterial compliance by novel advanced glycation end-product crosslink breaker. Circulation 2001;104: 1464–70.

General Principles of Hypertension Management in the Elderly

Mary V. Corrigan, MD[a,b,]*, Muralidhar Pallaki, MD[c,d]

KEYWORDS

• Geriatric • Hypertension • Elderly • Aging • Guideline

HTN is common and leads to significant adverse health outcomes, such as stroke, myocardial infarction, and renal insufficiency.[1] The geriatric population (defined as older than 65 years) comprises 13% of the population, and the "oldest old" (older than 85 years) are the largest growing segment of that group. Overall, HTN affects 65 million adults in the United States.[2] Within the elderly population, those older than 75 years have the highest rate of the condition. The prevalence of the condition is increasing, and blood pressure control rates remain poor. Almost two-thirds of those older than 60 years have HTN. Data from The Framingham study show that more than 90% of subjects older than 55 years who were normotensive at the start eventually become hypertensive.[3] HTN in the community nursing home population has been reported in up to 57% of men and 60% of women[4] and up to 71% of individuals in academic nursing homes.[5] Cardiovascular disease is the leading cause of death among elderly Americans. Stroke, heart failure, and premature death account for the associated morbidity and mortality with untreated and undertreated HTN.

The cardiovascular risk, morbidity, and mortality rise with age. The higher the systolic blood pressure and pulse pressure, (the difference between the systolic and diastolic) the higher the risk for morbidity and mortality due to cardiovascular events.

[a] Department of Family Practice, Case Western Reserve University School of Medicine, Cleveland, OH 44106, USA
[b] Section of Geriatrics, MetroHealth System, Senior Health and Wellness Center, Old Brooklyn Campus, 4229 Pearl Road, Cleveland, OH 44109, USA
[c] Case Western Reserve University School of Medicine, Cleveland, OH 44106, USA
[d] Section of Geriatrics, Louis Stokes Veterans Affairs Medical Center, 10701 East Boulevard, Cleveland, OH 44106, USA
* Corresponding author. Section of Geriatrics, MetroHealth System, Senior Health and Wellness Center, Old Brooklyn Campus, 4229 Pearl Road, Cleveland, OH 44109.
E-mail address: mcorrigan@metrohealth.org (M.V. Corrigan).

Clin Geriatr Med 25 (2009) 207–212
doi:10.1016/j.cger.2009.01.004
0749-0690/09/$ – see front matter © 2009 Published by Elsevier Inc.

geriatric.theclinics.com

The treatment of this condition has been shown in prospective, double-blind, placebo-controlled trials to decrease the incidence of adverse cardiovascular events 36% in older persons[3] and 34% in those older than 80 years.[4] Specifically, treatment reduced stroke risk by 34%, heart failure by 39%, and major cardiovascular events by 22%. Of note, an insignificant increase in all-cause mortality of treated individuals was 6%. Based on the known data, there is no threshold age above which treatment should be discontinued.[6]

DEFINITION OF HTN/ISH

A systolic pressure greater than 140 mm Hg and a diastolic pressure greater than 90 mm Hg noted on at least two visits during several weeks define HTN.[1]

Not only does the prevalence of HTN increase with age but its pattern also changes. After 50 years, isolated systolic HTN predominates. The diastolic pressure tends to fall as the systolic pressure increases. For every 20/10 mm Hg increase, cardiovascular risk roughly doubles. Notably, only 5% of the elderly have secondary HTN, the majority of which is renovascular in nature.[7]

PATHOGENESIS OF HTN

Atherosclerosis and decrease in elastin result in reduced compliance and elasticity of large arteries in the aged. This stiffening of the arteries underlies the pathology behind systolic HTN.[3] Total peripheral resistance is increased in the elderly, and age-related decrease in baroreceptor sensitivity exists. Because of this lack of baroreceptor sensitivity, the elderly experience greater fluctuations in their blood pressure. In addition, dysfunction in autoregulation exists in the target organs of the brain, heart, and kidney. Blood pressure has a circadian variation in the elderly. Blood pressure decreases while asleep and in the afternoon and is increased slightly in the evening and most pronounced in the early morning. The nighttime dip decreases with age and is nonexistent in many elderly men older than 80 years. This "nondipping" nocturnal state and the "morning surge" are both associated with increased risk of ischemic heart disease and cerebrovascular events.[7]

HTN TREATMENT GUIDELINES

The Seventh Report of the Joint National Committee on Detection, Evaluation, and Treatment of Hypertension (JNC 7) recommends that the goal of treatment of HTN in the elderly is to reduce the blood pressure to less than 140/90 mm Hg and to less than 130/80 mm Hg in older persons with diabetes mellitus or chronic renal insufficiency.[4] Likewise, treatment must look to lifestyle factors contributing to HTN as well as causes of elevated blood pressure, including noncompliance with medication, inadequate dosing of medications, and secondary causes.[8]

In 2006, the United States Preventive Services Task Force reaffirmed its 2003— Grade A recommendation to continue screening the elderly for HTN. The benefits of such screening outweighed any harm.[2]

SPECIAL POPULATIONS—OLDEST OLD AND NURSING HOME RESIDENTS

Studies of the oldest old, those with a mean age of 84 years and adequately treated for their high blood pressure, showed a decrease in stroke after 13 months.[3] Death from stroke is as high as 52% in individuals older than 80 years. Clearly, HTN is a major risk factor associated with stroke. In fact, a linear relationship exists between the two, although it is attenuated with age. The death rate reduction from stroke and the risk of stroke has been noted to decrease with treatment. Some studies show an actual decrease in death from any cause. Similarly, a large reduction in heart failure was noted in the Hypertension in the Very Elderly Trial.[9,10] Some trials suggest that the incidence of Alzheimer's dementia may be lower in the subset of elderly treated for HTN.[3]

One confounding factor is that a significant proportion of elders experience orthostatic hypotension, which makes the treatment of HTN tricky in light of their increased risk for falls.[11] Aged individuals also experience postprandial hypotension that needs to be taken into consideration when monitoring and treating blood pressure.[7]

ASSOCIATED PROBLEMS WITH HTN

Diabetes, hyperlipidemia, and HTN are often concomitant problems. Elderly individuals have decreased insulin sensitivity. The complications for elderly with these combined conditions are only compounded and point to the need for adequate treatment.[7] Obesity, especially central or abdominal obesity, incurs greater risk of HTN.[12]

PHARMACOLOGIC TREATMENT

One overriding geriatric principle is to avoid medications known to interfere with each other and to use the least possible number of medications to treat disease. Combination drugs may simplify treatment regimens, particularly in patients who have difficulty swallowing multiple pills. Polypharmacy is of concern as is achieving therapeutic endpoints as outlined in the JNC 7. Fixed-dose combination pills may be more cost effective by reducing the number of copays required. Safety, efficacy, and adherence are all considerations that must be weighted when prescribing combination medication. In general, starting with 1 medication at the lowest effective dose is suggested.[13]

The risk of underprescribing in the elderly, though, can lead to unnecessary adverse consequences. Therefore, a rational balance between polypharmacy and not treating needs to occur.[14,15] Of course, starting low and going slow are judicious when dealing with the frail elderly especially. Quality of life is an important consideration in making choices about the treatment of a chronic condition such as HTN.

More often than not, the elderly will require two or more medications to control their blood pressure. Diuretics are often the first-line choice. Medication choices are often dependent on the presence of other comorbid conditions.[3,8]

Geriatric Prescribing Guidelines

- Before adding additional medications to patients' drug regimen, their diagnosis should be confirmed.
- If feasible, only one medication would be changed at a time to assess the effects and response to that medication.
- When a patient does not respond to a medication, it is important to know whether the patient is taking the medication correctly.
- To increase compliance/adherence, the simplest effective treatment regimen should be prescribed. Many medications can be dosed once a day, and very few need them more than twice.
- Before adding additional agents, a single medication should be given adequate time at an effective dose to produce a therapeutic response.

- An important aspect of polypharmacy is drug-drug interactions. Drug-drug interactions are understandable and preventable if a clinician has a comprehensive list of a patients' medications.
- The patient should be educated on what kind of side effects the new medication may produce.
- Consider treatment alternatives, such as exercise and diet, before prescribing an additional medication.
- The patient's ability to pay for or otherwise obtain the medications should be considered when adding to the therapy.
- Before adding an additional medication to a complex patient, the frequency and duration of physician visits may need to be increased to allow for proper assessment of the patient's current medication regimen.

Implementation of nonpharmacologic techniques to lower blood pressure and the approach to patients with resistant HTN are important issues the clinician taking care of the elderly patient has to consider; these are detailed in other sections of this journal.

Barriers to treatment of HTN

Studies have also shown that elderly patients who have multiple medical problems are often undertreated, which is termed as "treatment inertia." Reports have shown that in more than 50% of patients with poorly controlled blood pressure, there have been no changes made in their medication regime by the physician.[8] Judgments are inaccurately made that treatment of the primary problem is sufficient often excluding HTN. In some situations, more medications are felt to be worse than the benefits they offer. In addition, patients may prefer fewer pills, despite their long-term efficacy.[14] Unfortunately, senior's prescription drug coverage is scant; more than 40% of Medicare enrollees have no benefit plan, which curtails the ability to afford more medication even if clinically indicated.[14]

SOLUTIONS TO INERTIA—CHRONIC DISEASE SELF-MANAGEMENT PROGRAMS

One approach to have shown benefit in effective treatment of HTN to target level in the elderly is the use of multidisciplinary teams composed of physicians, nurses, dieticians, and pharmacists. Including the patient in the care plan process has also been beneficial through education and reminders, such as the use of pill boxes.[16] Lifestyle modification with specific goals for changing diet and exercise works better than general advice.[17]

CLINICAL IMPLICATIONS, PRACTICAL ADVICE, AND PATIENT EDUCATION

Physicians also need to be educated in treating the geriatric population.[4] When measuring blood pressure, both arms should be used, and the higher of the two treated. Likewise, measurements should be taken in the standing and sitting position.[5] Cuffs must be the right size and properly calibrated. Once diagnosed with HTN, the physician should look for end organ damage by a comprehensive history, physical examination, and appropriate diagnostic testing.[18] Follow-up for the elderly who have reached target blood pressure should be every 3 to 6 months. Annual electrolytes should be obtained at a minimum. Ambulatory blood pressure monitoring is also useful in determining cases of white coat HTN.[19]

Quality of life is always a consideration in treatment of chronic conditions in the geriatric population. This includes life satisfaction, ability to perform one's instrumental and general activities of daily living, as well as one's outlook on life. Practitioners must also take into account patients suffering from depression and dementia. Clearly, negative outcomes from undertreatment of HTN, such as stroke, would have a huge impact on these quality-of-life indicators.[7]

SUMMARY

Despite the growing number of geriatric patients and the high prevalence of HTN, undertreatment of this condition still exists. Clearly, the cardiovascular and cerebrovascular complications can be decreased by treating to target. Through patient and physician education, this chronic malady can be treated with positive quality-of-life outcomes, even in the oldest old. As long as lifestyle and geriatric principles of prescribing are followed, inertia can change to action with satisfactory results for the aged patient.

REFERENCES

1. Wolff T, Miller T. Screening for high blood pressure: U.S. Preventive Services Task Force reaffirmation recommendation statement. Ann Intern Med 2007;147(11): 783–6.
2. Wolff T, Miller T. Evidence for the reaffirmation of the U.S. Preventive Services Task Force recommendation screening for high blood pressure. Ann Intern Med 2007; 147(11):787–91.
3. Chobaniian AV. Isolated systolic hypertension in the elderly. N Engl J Med 2007; 357:780–96.
4. Aronow WS. Drug therapy of older persons with hypertension [editorial]. J Am Med Dir Assoc March 2006;7:193–6.
5. Koka M, Joseph J, Aronow WS. Adequacy of Control of Hypertension in an Academic Nursing Home. J Am Med Dir Assoc 2007;8:538–40.
6. Cheng HY. Barriers for Underuse of Antihypertensive Drug Therapy for Nursing Home Residents with Hypertension [letters to the editor]. J Am Med Dir Assoc 2006;7:405–6.
7. Ogihara T, Hiwada K, Morimoto S, et al. Guidelines for treatment of hypertension in the elderly-2002 revised version. Hypertens Res 2003;26:1–36.
8. Moser M, Setaro JF. Resistant or difficult–to–control hypertension. N Engl J Med 2006;355:385–92.
9. Beckett NS, Peters R, Fletcher AE, et al. Treatment of hypertension in patients 80 years of age or older. N Engl J Med 2008;358(18):1887–98.
10. Cheng HY. The oldest old with hypertension: treat or not treat? J Am Geriatr Soc 2007;55(1):136–7.
11. Iwanczyk L, Weintraub NT, Rubenstein LZ. Orthostatic hypotension in the nursing home setting. J Am Med Dir Assoc 2006;7:163–7.
12. Hayashi T, Boyko EJ, Leonetti DL, et al. Fat content inside the abdomen helps predict whether Japanese Americans develop hypertension. Ann Intern Med 2004;140:992–1000.
13. Tangalos EG, Zarowitz BJ. Combination drug therapy. J Am Med Dir Assoc 2005; 6:406–9.
14. Rochan PA, Gurwitz JH. Prescribing for seniors: neither too much nor too little. JAMA 1999;282(2):113–5.
15. Phillips LS, Twombly JG. It's time to overcome clinical inertia. Ann Intern Med 2008;148(10):783–5.

16. Roumie CL, Basy TA, Greevy R, et al. The effect of educational reminders on blood pressure in veterans with hypertension. Ann Intern Med 2006;145:166–75.
17. Elmer PJ, Obarzanek E, Vollmer WM, et al. The effects of lifestyle changes on long-term blood pressure control. Ann Intern Med 2006;144:485–95.
18. Saliba D, Soloman D, Rubenstein L, et al. Quality indicators for the management of medical conditions in nursing home residents. J Am Med Dir Assoc 2004;5: 297–309.
19. Hoffman I. Isolated systolic hypertension in the elderly. N Engl J Med 2007; 357(22):2307–8.

Nonpharmacologic Management of Hypertension in the Elderly

Aparna Padiyar, MD

KEYWORDS

- Hypertension • Elderly • Lifestyle modification • DASH diet
- Behavioral modification • Low salt diet • TONE • Exercise

Increases in blood pressure during a patient's lifespan were once thought to be inextricably related to aging and, therefore, inevitable. However, secluded populations, such as cloistered nuns, or unacculturated societies, such as the San Bushmen in southern Africa, do not exhibit such elevations in blood pressure with age.[1] Furthermore, data suggest that peoples migrating from underdeveloped to more urban areas manifest increases in blood pressure more similar to those of the population of the urban area into which they are settling as compared with those of the rural population from which they came.[2] Although the pathophysiology of hypertension in aging populations is complex and multifactorial, its onset is likely heavily influenced by lifestyle and environmental factors.

The prohypertensive effects of urbanization are difficult to escape. In the United States, 90% of 55-year-old normotensives will have hypertension by the age of 75.[3] Excesses in dietary sodium, weight gain from increased caloric intake in the setting of physical inactivity, excessive alcohol intake, and psychological stress all contribute to the development of hypertension. Lifestyle modification has long been recognized as an essential component to the treatment of hypertension. The elderly population in particular, having seen the effects of hypertension, may be more motivated to pursue lifestyle change.

However, the vast majority of hypertensive patients in the United States receive suboptimal counseling regarding lifestyle modification, and this is particularly true of the elderly. Data from the National Ambulatory Medical Care Survey and the National Hospital Ambulatory Medical Care Survey for 1999 and 2000 revealed that for the 137 million patient encounters with a diagnosis of hypertension, nutrition and exercise counseling were provided at only 35% and 26% of visits, respectively.[4] Patients older

Division of Nephrology and Hypertension, Department of Medicine, Case Western Reserve University, University Hospitals-Case Medical Center, 11100 Euclid Avenue, Cleveland, OH 44106, USA
E-mail address: aparna.padiyar@uhhospitals.org

Clin Geriatr Med 25 (2009) 213–219
doi:10.1016/j.cger.2009.01.003
0749-0690/09/$ – see front matter © 2009 Elsevier Inc. All rights reserved.

than 74 years received the least nutrition (28%) and exercise (18%) counseling. This is an opportunity for improvement.

REDUCED SODIUM

Sodium excess plays a pivotal role in the pathophysiology underlying hypertension in the elderly. It has become increasingly clear that dietary salt intake and urinary salt excretion correlate both with elevated systolic blood pressure and pulse pressure.[5] A high-salt diet promotes profibrotic changes in vascular smooth muscle cells via induction of collagen synthesis. The resulting collagen deposition in the walls of large arteries leads to vessel stiffness and reduced compliance over time, a feature common in the isolated systolic hypertension so prevalent in older individuals.[6] Additionally, the decline in kidney function associated with aging predisposes older individuals to retain sodium to a greater extent than that in younger persons, contributing to a higher circulating blood volume.[7] A low-salt diet, therefore, may have a more pronounced benefit in the elderly, in whom decreased blood volume in the setting of decreased arterial compliance lends itself to greater reductions in blood pressure. Indeed, a meta-analysis of 56 randomized trials examining the effect of reduced dietary sodium on hypertension supports this hypothesis; blood pressure reductions were larger in trials of older hypertensive individuals.[8]

The most compelling evidence of the efficacy of dietary salt restriction in an aging population is the Trial of Nonpharmacologic Intervention in the Elderly (TONE).[9] The TONE investigators wished to test the hypothesis that dietary sodium restriction would allow safe withdrawal of pharmacologic therapy for hypertension. The study population consisted of 681 hypertensive patients aged 60 to 80 years who at baseline had a blood pressure less than 145/85 mm Hg while taking one antihypertensive medication. Patients were randomized to a low dietary salt intervention or to usual care, and after 3 months, the antihypertensive agent was withdrawn. Before medication withdrawal, the reduced sodium arm had a mean blood pressure reduction of 4.3 mm Hg systolic and 2.0 mm Hg diastolic ($P<.001$, $P = .001$). During a mean 27.8 months of follow-up, the primary endpoint—a composite of a rise in average BP to 150/90 mm Hg or more, the resumption of medication, or a cardiovascular event— occurred in 59% of reduced sodium group and 73% of control group participants (relative hazard ratio, 0.68, $P<.001$). The difference persisted regardless of race, gender, or weight, although it did not reach statistical significance in the very elderly (age group, 70–80 years)—perhaps a result of a small sample size. There appeared to be a dose-response effect, that is, greater sodium restriction was associated with less frequent occurrence of endpoints (P for trend, 0.002).

In an elderly patient population with a high dependence on prepackaged food and use of salt to compensate for diminished taste, the initial goal of the low-salt dietary intervention in TONE was ambitious. Investigators targeted a 24-hour dietary sodium intake of 80 mmol/L. Notably, this level is less than the Seventh Report of the Joint National Committee on Prevention, Detection, Evaluation and Treatment of High Blood Pressure (JNC VII) currently recommended upper limit of 100 mmol/L/d (2.4 g/d). To achieve this goal, TONE employed techniques using social acting theory to enhance understanding and achieve behavioral change. Nutritionists, experienced in lifestyle change techniques, used a combination of small group and individual meetings to advise participants on ways of changing eating patterns. In addition, they monitored individual and group progress at frequent intervals and helped participants adapt the lifestyle recommendations to their individual circumstances. The intervention was successful in reducing overall urinary sodium excretion by 40 mmol/d ($P = .001$).[10]

In sum, TONE demonstrated that a reduction in dietary sodium of 40 mmol/d in an elderly population results in approximately 30% decrease in the need for antihypertensive medication. Simply by changing food production and procurement procedures in senior centers, retirement communities, as well as meal-delivery programs, a passive decrease in sodium intake targeted for a large population of older patients is possible. More widespread access to dietary- and behavioral-intervention counseling programs would help to facilitate more aggressive sodium restriction and hypertension control.

DASH DIET

The lowest average blood pressures in an industrialized country have been found among a population of strict vegetarians in Massachusetts. Adhering to "macrobiotics," these individuals consume almost no animal products and instead rely upon whole grains, green leafy vegetables, squash, and root vegetables.[11] Since then, a number of studies have realized that a high intake of fruit and vegetables is associated with decreases not only in blood pressure and in change of blood pressure with age but also in overall cardiovascular risk.[12] The landmark DASH trial took its cue from such epidemiologic observations and established that a diet rich in fruits, vegetables, and low-fat dairy products with reduced saturated and total fat can lower blood pressure, independent of sodium restriction or weight loss.[13] Blood pressure reductions of 11.4/5.5 mm Hg were seen in hypertensive patients and 3.5/2.1 mm Hg in normotensive individuals after 8 weeks of dietary modification. Significant declines in blood pressure were observed in all population subgroups studied — including older patients (defined as age > 45 years) — but were particularly prominent in African Americans.[14] In combination with a low-sodium diet, even greater blood pressure reductions are possible.[15]

ALCOHOL

Alcohol has little effect on blood pressure unless taken chronically in large amounts. Although people older than 65 years generally consume less alcohol than do younger people, the extent of alcohol use in the elderly is a matter of some debate.[16] High rates of alcoholism in the older population have been found among surveys conducted in health care settings: Of elderly patients admitted to hospitals, 6% to 11% exhibit symptoms of alcoholism, and so do 20% of elderly patients in psychiatric wards, and 14% of elderly patients in emergency rooms.[17] Hospital staff are significantly less likely to recognize alcoholism in an older patient than in a younger patient, as the alcohol-related consequences of drinking are often mistaken for medical or psychiatric conditions common in the elderly.[18] The problem is confounded by the fact that questionnaires developed to screen for alcoholism are ineffective in this population, who may not exhibit the social, legal, and occupational consequences of alcohol misuse generally used to diagnose problem drinkers.

With regard to hypertension treatment, JNC VII guidelines suggest limiting alcohol consumption to less than 1 oz (30 mL) of ethanol, 24 oz (720 mL) beer, 10 oz (300 mL) wine, or 2 oz (60 mL) 100-proof whiskey in hypertensive men or 1/2 oz daily ethanol in women.

PHYSICAL ACTIVITY AND WEIGHT LOSS

The pervasive relationship that exists among obesity, hypertension, and cardiovascular morbidity is a well-recognized phenomenon. Systolic blood pressure rises 3.0 mm Hg, and diastolic 2.3 mm Hg, for each 10 kg increase in body weight; each 10 kg increase in body weight is also associated with a 12% increase in coronary heart disease risk and 24% increase in the risk of stroke.[19,20] This relationship clearly extends to the elderly. Furthermore, regular aerobic exercise has been shown not only to reduce blood pressure but also to improve overall cardiovascular health, a finding that has been replicated in studies of geriatric cohorts.[21,22]

The second tier of the TONE (see above) examined the effect of modest physical activity and subsequent weight loss on blood pressure control.[9] A total of 585 obese participants (body mass index, $\geq$27.8 kg/m^2 for men and $\geq$27.3 kg/m^2 for women), with blood pressure less than 145/85 mm Hg while taking one antihypertensive, were randomized to one of four groups: sodium restriction or weight loss alone, sodium restriction and weight loss combined, or usual care. After 3 months, the anti-hypertensive agent was withdrawn, and the patients followed to trial completion (approximately 2 years) or to occurrence of the primary endpoint (again, a composite of a rise in average BP to 150/90 mm Hg or more, the resumption of medication, or a cardiovascular event). Compared with usual care, hazard ratios were 0.60 (95% CI, 0.45–0.80; P<.001) for reduced sodium intake alone, 0.64 (95% CI, 0.49–0.85; P = .002) for weight loss alone, and 0.47 (95% CI, 0.35–0.64; P<.001) for the combination of reduced sodium intake and weight loss.

The goal of the weight loss intervention was to achieve and maintain a weight loss of 4.5 kg (10 lb) or greater. Again, TONE used exercise counselors, experienced in lifestyle change techniques, to oversee a combination of small group and individual meetings. The average reduction in weight was approximately 3.5 to 4.5 kg (P<.001) versus an average 0.9-kg reduction (95% CI, 0.4–1.3) for those not assigned to weight loss. Interestingly, the mean weight loss was 1.0 kg (95% CI, -0.1–2.0 kg) greater in those assigned to weight loss alone than in those assigned to sodium reduction and weight loss combined.

By reducing average body weight about 3.5 kg, patients decreased their need for antihypertensives more than 30%. Notably, the patients assigned to the combined intervention group were the most successful in maintaining good blood pressure control off medication. Moreover, the effect persisted.[23] At 4 years, after the end of TONE and discontinuation of contact of the participants with the clinical center, 23% of the combined intervention group versus 7% in the usual care group were still off medication (P = .012).

How realistic are the physical activity and weight loss goals of the TONE trial? Inactivity tends to increase with age, as only 30% of patients older than 65 years report participation in regular physical activity.[24] Multiple barriers exist when counseling elderly patients to exercise, both physician and patient centered. Patient concerns over health, self-image, limited space, and time as well as physician concerns over safety, exercise tolerance, and lack of perceived effect are all issues that need to be addressed. However, a physician's recommendation to increase physical activity can be a strong motivator to patients. Behavioral counseling by other members of the health care team may be beneficial. Establishment of realistic goals that take into account patient needs and preferences, with opportunities for reinforcement, seems to be most efficacious.

Weight loss has been found to be a predictor of hip fracture among women aged 65 years or older by the Study of Osteoporotic Factors Research Group.[25] Although it is unclear if these findings apply to structured weight loss programs that include increased physical activity, calcium and vitamin D supplementation may be prudent.

COMBINATION INTERVENTION

Combinations of interventions may be particularly effective in the management of hypertension in the elderly. The multicenter PREMIER[26] trial tested the effect c multicomponent lifestyle interventions on blood pressure. This ambitious study randomized 810 individuals (average age, 50 years) with prehypertension to stage 1 hypertension to one of three groups: (1) an "advice-only" group that met with a nutritional counselor once to discuss general principles of weight loss, sodium restriction, physical activity, and the DASH diet; (2) a behavioral intervention that implemented established recommendations of 100 mEq daily sodium restriction, alcohol moderation, prescribed 180 min/wk moderate-intensity physical activity, and 6.8 kg weight loss (Established [Est]); and (3) the same established recommendations plus DASH diet (Est plus DASH). After 6 months, all groups saw a decrease in the initial hypertension prevalence of 38%, to 26% in the advice-only group, 17% in the established group ($P = .01$ compared with that in the advice-only group), and 12% in the Est plus DASH group ($P<.001$ compared with that in the advice-only group; $P = .12$ compared with that in the established group). The mean reduction in systolic blood pressure was 3.7 mm Hg ($P<.001$) in the established group and 4.3 mm Hg ($P<.001$) in the established plus DASH group. Both the Est and Est Plus DASH interventions caused statistically significant blood pressure reductions in individuals older than and younger than 50 years. Notably, the effect in the Est Plus DASH group was significantly more pronounced in older individuals.

PSYCHOLOGICAL STRESS

Depression and anxiety have previously been associated with development of hypertension.[27] Whether this correlation carries over into an elderly patient population is not clear. The Three-City Study was a cross-sectional investigation of 9,294 individuals aged 65 years and older, living at home, in 3 French cities (Bordeaux, Dijon, and Montpellier).[28] Overall, 31% of participants met the criteria for depression, and 77.5% had hypertension. Lower blood pressure values were found in depressive individuals compared with those in nondepressive ones, in both men (systolic, 148.2 vs 151.8 mm Hg, $P<.002$; diastolic, 83.0 vs 84.7 mm Hg, $P = .003$) and women (systolic, 141.7 vs 144.7 mm Hg, $P<.0001$; diastolic, 80.7 vs 81.4 mm Hg, $P<.02$). These associations were independent of the use of antihypertensive or psychotropic medications.

In another cross-sectional study, this time of 2,564 Mexican Americans aged 65 years or older, a positive emotion score was significantly associated with lower blood pressure.[29] It is unknown if interventions targeting the emotional health of older adults might be efficacious in the prevention or treatment of hypertension.

Table 1 Goals of behavioral modification to treat hypertension in the elderly	
Low-salt diet	80–100 mmol/d[9]
DASH diet	Diet rich in fruits, vegetables, and low-fat dairy products with reduced saturated and total fat[13]
Physical activity	180 min/wk moderate-intensity physical activity[26]
Weight loss	3.5–4.5 kg[8]
Moderation of alcohol	<1 oz (30 mL) of ethanol, 24 oz (720 mL) beer, 10 oz (300 mL) wine, or 2 oz (60 mL) 100-proof whiskey in men or 1/2 oz daily ethanol in women per JNC VII recommendations

A combination of the above interventions results in greater antihypertensive effect.[8,23,26]

SUMMARY

Nonpharmacologic lifestyle modifications are effective in the management of hypertension in the elderly, particularly when used in combination (**Table 1**). The lack of use of these techniques and the motivation of elderly patients to pursue lifestyle changes provides tremendous opportunity for improvement. Dietary salt restriction, the DASH diet, moderation of alcohol consumption, physical activity, and weight loss can all be incorporated successfully into the management of elderly hypertensive patients and indeed should be considered the cornerstone of therapy. Lifestyle interventions not only reduce blood pressure, prevent, or delay the development of hypertension and enhance the efficacy of antihypertensive medications but also decrease cardiovascular risk.

REFERENCES

1. Timio M, Verdecchia P, Venanzi S, et al. Age and blood pressure changes. A 20-year follow-up study in nuns in a secluded order. Hypertension 1988;12: 457–61.
2. Poulter NR, Khaw K, Hopwood BE, et al. Determinants of blood pressure changes due to urbanization: a longitudinal study. J Hypertens Suppl 1985;3(3):S375–7.
3. Vasan RS, Beiser A, Seshadri S, et al. Residual lifetime risk for developing hypertension in middle-aged women and men: The Framingham Heart Study. JAMA 2002;287:1003–10.
4. Mellen PB, Palla SL, Goff DC, et al. Prevalence of nutrition and exercise counseling for patients with hypertension United States, 1999 to 2000. J Gen Intern Med 2004;19(9):917–24.
5. Stamler J, Rose G, Stamler R, et al. INTERSALT study findings. Public health and medical care implications. Hypertension 1989;14:570–7.
6. Simon G. Pathogenesis of structural vascular changes in hypertension. J Hypertens 2004;22:3–10.
7. Luft FC, Weinberger MH, Fineberg NS, et al. Effects of age on renal sodium homeostasis and its relevance to sodium sensitivity. Am J Med 1987;82:9–15.
8. Midgley JP, Matthew AG, Greenwood CM, et al. Effect of reduced dietary sodium on blood pressure: a meta-analysis of randomized controlled trials. JAMA 1996; 275:1590–7.
9. Appel LJ, Espeland MA, Easter L, et al. Effects of reduced sodium intake on hypertension control in older individuals results from the Trial of Nonpharmacologic Interventions in the Elderly (TONE). Arch Intern Med 2001;161:685–93.
10. Whelton PK, Appel LJ, Espeland MA, et al. Sodium reduction and weight loss in the treatment of hypertension in older persons. A randomised controlled trial of non-pharmacological interventions in the elderly (TONE). JAMA 1998;279: 839–46.
11. Sacks FM, Kass EH. Low blood pressure in vegetarians: effects of specific foods and nutrients. Am J Clin Nutr 1988;48:795–800.
12. Bazzano KA, He J, Ogden LG, et al. Fruit and vegetable intake and risk of cardiovascular disease in US adults: the First National Health and Nutrition Examination Survey epidemiologic follow-up study. Am J Clin Nutr 2002;76:93–9.
13. Appel LJ, Moore TJ, Obarzanek E, et al. A clinical trial of the effects of dietary patterns on blood pressure. N Engl J Med 1997;336:1117–24.
14. Svetkey LP, Simons-Morton D, Vollmer WM, et al. Effects of dietary patterns on blood pressure subgroup analysis of the Dietary Approaches to Stop Hypertension (DASH) randomized clinical trial. Arch Intern Med 1999;159:285–93.

15. Sacks FM, Svetkey LP, Vollmer WM, et al. Effects on blood pressure of reduced dietary sodium and the Dietary Approaches To Stop Hypertension (DASH) diet. N Engl J Med 2001;344(1):3–10.
16. National Institute On Alcohol Abuse And Alcoholism. Alcohol alert, No. 40, April 1998. Updated. Bethesda (MD): The Institute; 2000.
17. Council on Scientific Affairs, American Medical Association. Alcoholism in the elderly. JAMA 1996;275(10):797–801.
18. Curtis JR, Geller G, Stokes EJ, et al. Characteristics, diagnosis, and treatment of alcoholism in elderly patients. J Am Geriatr Soc 1989;37:310–6.
19. National Heart, Lung and Blood Institute Initiative Expert Panel on the Identification, Evaluation and Treatment of Overweight and Obesity in Adults. Clinic guidelines on the identification, evaluation, and treatment of overweight and obesity in adults. The evidence report. NIH. NHLBI. Obes Res 1998;6:51s–209s.
20. Stanton JA, Lowenthal DT. The evidence for lifestyle modification in lowering blood pressure in the elderly. Am J Geriatr Cardiol 2000;9(1):27–33.
21. Seals DR, Silverman HG, Reiling MJ, et al. Effect of regular aerobic exercise on elevated blood pressure in postmenopausal women. Am J Cardiol 1997;80:49–55.
22. Braith RW, Pollock MI, Lowenthal DT, et al. Moderate and high intensity exercise lowers blood pressure in nomotensive subjects 60–79 years of age. Am J Cardiol 1994;73:1124–8.
23. Kostis JB, Wilson AC, Shindler DM, et al. Persistence of normotension after discontinuation of lifestyle intervention in the trial of TONE. Trial of Nonpharmacologic Interventions in the Elderly. Am J Hypertens 2002;15(8):732–4.
24. Heath JM, Stuart MR. Prescribing exercise for frail elders. J Am Board Fam Pract 2002;15:218–28.
25. Ensrud KE, Cauley J, Lipschutz R, et al. Weight change and fractures in older women. Study of Osteoporotic Fractures Research Group. Arch Intern Med 1997;157(8):857–63.
26. Writing Group of the PREMIER Collaborative Research Group. Effects of comprehensive lifestyle modification on blood pressure control, main results of the PREMIER Clinical Trial. JAMA 2003;289:2083–93.
27. Jonas BS, Lando JF. Negative affect as a prospective risk factor for hypertension. Psychosom Med 2000;62:188–96.
28. Lenoir H, Lacombe JM, Dufouil C, et al. Relationship between blood pressure and depression in the elderly. The Three-City Study. J Hypertens 2008;26(9):1765–72.
29. Ostir GV, Berges IM, Markides KS, et al. Hypertension in older adults and the role of positive emotions. Psychosom Med 2006;68(5):727–33.

Polypharmacy in the Elderly: Focus on Drug Interactions and Adherence in Hypertension

Danielle Cooney, PharmD, BC-ADM*, Kristina Pascuzzi, PharmD, BCPS

KEYWORDS

- Polypharmacy • Adherence • Hypertension • Medication
- Elderly • Geriatric

The pathophysiology of hypertension (HTN) in the elderly is multifactorial; it is characterized by increase in total peripheral vascular resistance (PVR), decreased compliance of the large middle arteries, tendency toward a decrease in cardiac output and circulating blood volume, increased lability of blood pressure (BP) due to age-related baroreceptor function, decreased blood flow, and dysfunction of the autoregulation process in the kidneys, heart, and brain. These changes can make treating HTN in the elderly challenging, putting patients at increased risk of developing adverse events and complications with antihypertensive medications. Therefore, caution must be taken when initiating and titrating medications for HTN in the elderly.[1]

ALTERED PHARMACOKINETICS AND PHARMACODYNAMICS IN THE ELDERLY

There has been no clinical definition of age that has been reliably associated with age-related changes in drug pharmacokinetics or pharmacodynamics.[2] There are many physiologic changes that occur with aging, some of which can affect a person's response to antihypertensive medications.[3] Age-related changes that affect body composition or function include, but are not limited to, decreased renal function, decreased hepatic blood flow, decreased albumin, increased body fat, decreased lean muscle mass, and decreased total body water.

Department of Pharmacy, Louis Stokes Veterans Affairs Medical Center, Pharmacy Service (119W), 10701 East Blvd, Cleveland, OH 44106, USA
* Corresponding author.
E-mail address: danielle.corwin@va.gov (D. Cooney).

Clin Geriatr Med 25 (2009) 221–233
doi:10.1016/j.cger.2009.01.005
0749-0690/09/$ – see front matter. Published by Elsevier Inc.

geriatric.theclinics.com

Absorption

Age-related changes in gastrointestinal function include increased gastric pH, delayed gastric emptying, and impaired intestinal motility. Although these changes occur, the extent of drug absorption is not often altered in the elderly.[4]

Distribution

Distribution of medications can be affected by changes in body composition and changes in protein binding. As stated above, the elderly usually have an increase in adipose tissue, decrease in lean body mass, and reduction in total body water. These alterations can cause significant changes in the volume of distribution of various medications. For water-soluble drugs, the reduced volume of distribution can increase the initial concentration in the central compartment and cause higher plasma concentrations. On the other hand, for lipid-soluble drugs, the larger volume of distribution can lead to prolonged half-lives and duration of action. The elderly tend to have a decreased albumin and increased alpha$_1$ acid glycoprotein levels. These changes can make the elderly more susceptible to acute effects of multiple drug therapy when highly protein-bound drugs are prescribed together. As the body ages, cardiac output is often reduced and PVR increases, leading to a decrease in total systemic perfusion of the vital organs including the kidneys and liver. This reduction in perfusion can decrease the body's ability to metabolize and excrete medications.

Metabolism

Changes in drug metabolism can lead to elevated drug responses in elderly patients. Drug metabolism, which mainly occurs in the liver, is dependent on hepatic function and hepatic blood flow. The elderly have approximately 40% decrease in the hepatic blood flow compared with someone who is 25 years old.[5] This results in a major reduction of first-pass metabolism of drugs. Medications subject to oxidative phase I metabolism exhibit decreased elimination. This is because phase I metabolism is catalyzed by the cytochrome P450 (CYP 450) system in the smooth endoplasmic reticulum of the hepatocytes, a process that decreases with age. Some antihypertensive medications that are affected by this first-pass metabolism include propranolol, verapamil, and nifedipine. One study found that the average clearance of propranolol declined from 13.2 mL/min/kg in young adults to 7.8 mL/min/kg in the elderly, whereas the oral bioavailability increases from 0.3 to 0.55, respectively.[6] Phase II metabolism, which involves the conjugation of a drug molecule by glucuronidation, acetylation, or sulfation, is not generally affected by age.[7] One must also take into account the increased likelihood that older patients will take a medication that inhibits or induces the metabolism of their other medications. The CYP 450 system is responsible for the metabolism of many medications in the liver. The CYP 450 enzymes involved in most drug interactions are 3A4, 2D6, 1A2, and 2C9. Some common antihypertensives that are metabolized by CYP 3A4 include metoprolol, propranolol, amlodipine, and nifedipine. If a potent CYP 3A4 inhibitor, such as amiodarone, erythromycin, or specific antifungals, is prescribed to an elderly patient on one of the antihypertensives listed above, a potentially serious drug interaction with toxicity could occur.

Elimination

Renal function progressively declines with advanced age, and having HTN can accelerate this decline in renal function. Renal blood flow is reduced by approximately 1% per year after 50 years.[7] The decline in renal function is not accurately reflected by an increase in serum creatinine in the elderly due to the decline in muscle mass. Creatinine is a product of muscle breakdown, and because of a decreased muscle mass with aging, production of creatinine is reduced. The commonly used Cockcroft-Gault equation may overestimate renal function, especially in the very frail, emaciated, elderly patients. Since many medications have a renal mode of elimination, a reduction in renal function can affect the elimination of a drug if it is more than 60% excreted by the kidneys. Higher blood levels of a medication whose elimination is primarily renal are found when the glomerular filtration rate declines. This can result in accumulation of the medication, producing higher drug levels for prolonged periods of time. One common antihypertensive medication that is primarily renally eliminated is atenolol.[8] The half-life of atenolol can be significantly increased in patients with renal insufficiency. In patients with varying degrees of renal insufficiency, the half-life can range from 10 to 28 hours but can be up to 100 hours. Urinary excretion in 24 hours can be declined to 29% of the dose administered.[9] The manufacturer for atenolol indicates that in patients with a creatinine clearance of 35 mL/min or greater, usual doses of atenolol may be administered, since no significant accumulation is expected. For patients with creatinine clearances between 15 and 35 mL/min, the maximum recommended dosage should not exceed 50 mg/d. In patients with severe renal insufficiency (creatinine clearance less than 15 mL/min), the maximum recommended dosage is 25 mg/d.[10]

PHARMACODYNAMICS IN THE ELDERLY

Pharmacodynamics is the physiologic or psychological response to a drug. Compared with pharmacokinetics, less is known about pharmacodynamic changes in the elderly. The changes in drug pharmacodynamics can arise from changes in receptor number, receptor affinity, postreceptor effects, receptor membrane interactions, structural changes in organs and tissues, and altered homeostatic functions.

Age-related changes can be separated into autonomic nervous system and central nervous system (CNS) changes. In the autonomic nervous system, elderly patients have a reduction in β adrenergic receptor activity in the cardiovascular system and respiratory tract. As a result, the elderly may be less responsive to β adrenergic blockers (such as atenolol, metoprolol, and propranolol) and to β adrenergic agonists (such as formoterol and salmeterol). The total number of β receptors does not change in the elderly; it is the postreceptor events that occur after receptor activation that are altered, thus reducing the ability to activate adenylate cyclase. The altered postreceptor events have been attributed to altered intracellular conditions.[4] The CNS changes are memory impairment and decreased ability to process new information. This could affect a patient's adherence to medications and ability to understand the correct instructions for a new medication.

The hallmark of the aging process in physiologic terms is diminished adaptive capacity. Physiologic responses that require the integrated ability of several organ systems may result in a slow recovery rate in the elderly patient. One example of this is the homeostatic response with postural hypotension. The elderly have impaired baroreceptor reflex activity due to reduced sensitivity or function of the carotid sinus and aortic arch baroreceptors and reduced cardiac response to stimulation. This makes the elderly more likely to have exaggerated postural changes in BP that are not compensated by a reflex increase in cardiac output.[11]

DRUG INTERACTIONS

These age-related changes in body composition and function can make the elderly more susceptible to medication interactions. The potential for drug-drug interactions increases with rising age, because the elderly typically receive a larger amount of medications and also because the renal elimination of medications may be reduced. One study showed the impact that the number of medications can have on drug interactions. Approximately 13% of patients on two medications developed a medication interaction, which increased to 82% of patients when the number of medications taken increased to six or more.[12] A list of agents that interact by either increasing or decreasing the antihypertensive effect of BP medications is summarized in **Table 1**. Not included in the table is the risk of potentiating hypotension with the additive use of two or more antihypertensive medications. **Table 2** lists the most relevant interactions involving common antihypertensive medications. It is important to keep these in mind when initiating new therapies. There are several mechanisms in which medications can interact with others. There are pharmacokinetic interactions involving absorption, distribution, metabolism, and elimination. An example of a pharmacokinetic interaction would be the rise in plasma level and toxicity of digoxin that is provoked by verapamil. Another example would be how thiazide diuretics may decrease the renal elimination of lithium, possibly leading to toxic lithium levels. There are also pharmacodynamic interactions that can result in additive toxicity. A common antihypertensive example could be the use of a nondihydropyridine (DHP) calcium channel blocker such as verapamil in conjunction with

Table 1 Antihypertensive effects with interacting medications[1]		
	Agents that *Increase* Antihypertensive Effect	**Agents that *Decrease* Antihypertensive Effect**
Beta Blockers	Cimetidine Quinidine, fluoxetine, paroxetine (for those metabolized in the liver) Phenothiazines	NSAIDs Rifamycins, phenobarbital, tobacco (for those metabolized in the liver) Antacids (aluminum and calcium salts)
Calcium channel blockers	Cimetidine Macrolide antibiotics, antifungal azoles (with felodipine and nifedipine) Grapefruit juice (verapamil) Cyclosporine (with DHPs) Protease inhibitors (non-DHPs)	St John's wart: reduce diltiazem Rifampin Phenytoin Rifamycins Barbiturates Carbamazepine (Non-DHPs)
ACE-I and ARB	Diuretics Chlorpromazine	NSAIDs Antacids Aprotinin High-dose salicylates
Diuretics	—	NSAIDs Steroids Cholestyramine and Colestipol: with thiazides Aliskiren: with loops Phenytoin: with loops
Alpha blockers	Phosphodiesterase 5 inhibitors	NSAIDs

Abbreviations: ACE-I, angiotensin-converting enzyme inhibitors; ARB, angiotensin receptor blockers; DHP, dihydropyridine; NSAIDs, nonsteroidal anti-inflammatory drugs.

Data from Ogihara T, Hiwada K, Morimoto S, et al. Guidelines for treatment of hypertension in the elderly—2002 revised version. Hypertens Res 2003;26(1):26.

Table 2 Drug interactions with antihypertensives[1]	
Antihypertensive	**Drug Interactions**
Beta blockers	Antihyperglycemics: masks hypoglycemia Digoxin: bradycardia with propranolol Antiarrhythmics: decrease cardiac function, arrhythmias, and conduction defects Pseudoephedrine: increase in BP Phosphodiesterase 5 inhibitors: drop in BP Methacholine: enhanced toxic effects with metoprolol Acetylcholinesterase inhibitors: enhance bradycardic effects
Calcium channel blockers	Digoxin, carbamazepine, midazolam, ranolazine, risperidone: rise in blood levels with Non-DHPs Amiodarone: AV block and cardiac arrest with Non-DHPs Theophylline: levels increased with Non-DHPs Simvastatin and lovastatin: levels increased with Non-DHPs Cyclosporine, tacrolimus: increased blood levels Lithium: neurotoxic effects with Non-DHPs Carbamazepine: increased levels with diltiazem Buspirone: increased levels with Non-DHPs
ACE-I and ARB	Potassium supplements, potassium sparing diuretics, and trimethoprim: hyperkalemia NSAIDs: decrease renal function, hyperkalemia Lithium: increased levels Allopurinol: increase in sensitivity Loop diuretics: increased risk of hypovolemia Insulin: hypoglycemia Cyclosporine: enhanced nephrotoxic effects
Diuretics	Aminoglycosides: increase toxicity to kidneys with loop diuretics Lithium: rise in blood levels Antihyperglycemics: effects decreased with thiazides Neuromuscular blocking agents: prolonged action with thiazides Digoxin: diuretic-induced hypokalemia may predispose to toxicity Calcitriol: increased hypercalcemic effect with thiazides

Abbreviations: ACE-I, angiotensin-converting enzyme inhibitors; ARB, angiotensin receptor blockers; BP, blood pressure; Non-DHP, Nondihydropyridine; NSAIDs, Nonsteroidal anti-inflammatory drugs.

Data from Ogihara T, Hiwada K, Morimoto S, et al. Guidelines for treatment of hypertension in the elderly—2002 revised version. Hypertens Res 2003;26(1):26.

a beta blocker such as metoprolol, thus resulting in additive impairment of cardiac atrioventricular conduction and bradycardia. Some medications can directly affect BP regardless of any interacting medication. **Table 3** lists several common agents that have been shown to increase BP.

BEERS CRITERIA

Because of the pharmacokinetic and pharmacodynamic changes in the elderly, they are more prone to adverse drug reactions. Fick and colleagues[13] updated the Beers criteria in 2003, which is a publication that includes potentially inappropriate medications for use in the elderly, listed in two different formats. One table contains the potentially inappropriate medications *independent* of diagnoses or conditions, whereas the second table takes into account various diagnoses or conditions that could affect drug selection.[13] Included in this list are several

Table 3 Medications that can increase blood pressure[35,37]	
Medications	Mechanism of Action
NSAIDs	Sodium and fluid retention, decreased prostaglandin formation
Sympathomimetics	Vasoconstriction by blocking alpha receptors
Corticosteroids	Sodium retention
Erythropoietin	Increased blood viscosity
Cyclosporine	Renal vasoconstriction and sodium retention
Amphetamines	Increased catecholamines
Ergot alkaloids	Vasoconstriction
Anabolic steroids	Sodium retention

Abbreviation: NSAIDs, nonsteroidal anti-inflammatory drugs.

Data from Onusko E. Diagnosing secondary hypertension. Am Fam Physician 2003;68(1):42 and Chobanian AV, Bakris GL, Black HR, et al, and the National High Blood Pressure Education Program Coordinating Committee. The Seventh Report of the Joint National Committee on Prevention, Detection, Evaluation, and Treatment of High Blood Pressure. The JNC 7 report. JAMA 2003;289:2560–72.

classes of antihypertensive medications that need to be used with caution or generally avoided in the elderly.

ANTIHYPERTENSIVE MEDICATION THERAPY

Alpha$_1$ blockers are a class of BP medications that should be used with caution in the elderly.[13] Doxazosin (Cardura) is specifically listed in the Beers criteria as deemed inappropriate independent of the patient's other diagnoses or conditions.[13] The worrisome adverse effects from the alpha$_1$ blockers include syncope, postural hypotension, and, specifically, the "first-dose" effect. This class is often attractive for use because of its Food and Drug Administration-approved indication for the treatment of benign prostatic hyperplasia (BPH). Since BPH tends to be a condition associated with aging, potentially using one medication to treat two different conditions is appealing, as it can reduce pill burden as well as out-of-pocket medication expense for the patient. Alpha$_1$ blockers are not recommended as initial therapy for HTN based on the results of the Antihypertensive and Lipid-Lowering Treatment to Prevent Heart Attack (ALLHAT) Trial showing increased risk of heart failure (HF) compared to chlorthalidone.[14] If alpha$_1$ blockers are chosen for treatment in the elderly, the following points should be taken into consideration:

- Does the patient also have a diagnosis of BPH?
- Start with the lowest dose and titrate slowly, waiting at least 1 to 2 weeks between dosage adjustments[15]
- If the product being used is dosed once daily, instruct the patient to take it at bedtime
- Educate patient/caregiver about the potential adverse effects, specifically, orthostatic hypotension

As a class, beta blockers have many indications, including, but not limited to, HTN and HF. Many elderly patients will also carry a HF diagnosis, warranting the use of beta blockers. Various beta blockers have been used in the HTN trials specifically targeting the elderly population.[16–19] Propranolol is the only beta blocker listed on the Beers criteria.[13] Its use should be assessed when a patient has concomitant chronic obstructive pulmonary disease, for concern of causing bronchospasm. Since propranolol is a nonselective and highly lipophilic beta blocker, choosing a more selective and more hydrophilic beta blocker can reduce the potential for this adverse effect.[20] Atenolol and metoprolol are 2 commonly used beta blockers considered safe for treating HTN in the elderly, when BP and pulse are monitored. These medications need to be dosed according to the patient's renal or hepatic function.

Calcium channel blockers are another commonly used antihypertensive class of medications. Short-acting nifedipine is the only calcium channel blocker specifically listed on the Beers criteria and no longer has a role in the treatment of HTN.[13] However, the extended-release agents are commonly used.[21] To avoid hypotension, consider starting at the lowest dose and slowly titrating until target BP is achieved. With the elderly already prone to constipation, they should be educated about this potential adverse effect before initiating two specific agents in this class, verapamil and diltiazem. Nonpharmacologic approaches could be suggested to prevent this adverse effect from occurring, such as adequate fiber and fluid intake, as well as exercise.[22]

Medications acting on the CNS, including reserpine, methyldopa, and clonidine, all appear on the Beers list,[13] making them potentially inappropriate for use in the elderly. Reserpine exerts its pharmacologic effect by centrally depleting norepinephrine and dopamine.[21] Some concerns with this agent include sedation, and once doses exceed 0.25 mg daily, depression, impotence, and orthostatic hypotension can occur.[21] Clonidine works by stimulating alpha 2 adrenoreceptors, resulting in reduced sympathetic outflow from the CNS, producing a decrease in peripheral resistance, renal vascular resistance, heart rate, and BP. Orthostatic hypotension and CNS adverse effects (drowsiness, 35%; dizziness, 16%) are concerns when using clonidine.[23] Methyldopa works similar to clonidine in the CNS and has additional adverse effects, which include bradycardia and possible exacerbation of depression in the elderly. These agents are not used as first line for the treatment of HTN. However, if all other options have been exhausted, one of these medications may become necessary for treatment.

Although angiotensin-converting enzyme inhibitors (ACE-I) and angiotensin receptor blockers (ARB) are not included in the Beers criteria,[13] caution is still advised when prescribing these agents in the elderly population. ACE-I and ARB have many useful indications. Besides BP lowering, they can be used in HF, after having a myocardial infarction, or for their renoprotective effects. Many geriatric patients often have concomitant disease states, which make choosing one of these agents to treat HTN very beneficial. Since ACE-I and ARB are known to affect potassium and serum creatinine levels, close monitoring should be practiced when using them, especially after initiation and after any dosage increase.

Aside from the prescription medications mentioned previously, there are several nonprescription agents that also should be used with caution when managing BP in the elderly. Over-the-counter (OTC) medications, vitamins, and herbal products are widely available and easily accessible to the general population. As new drug entities are developed and brought to market, and as more products become available OTC, self-medication becomes increasingly more likely.[24] One study which assessed OTC use was the SLONE survey. Overall, 40% of study participants took a vitamin and/or mineral product and 14% took an herbal or other supplement.[24] Of the study participants, approximately 23% of them were aged 65 or older, which highlights how even the elderly population do self-medicate. Since these products are not benign and can potentially interact with prescription medications or exacerbate chronic conditions, clinicians need to specifically inquire about their use. Because a prescription is not needed before purchasing these agents, many patients do not look at these as "medicine," which is one reason why more intense questioning is often needed. The categories of these products specifically listed on the Beers criteria[13] affecting BP include decongestants, diet pills, and nonsteroidal anti-inflammatory drugs (NSAIDs). Decongestants are of concern as they can produce elevations in BP due to vasoconstriction. Even though pseudoephedrine has been replaced by phenylephrine in all OTC products available on US shelves, the possibility of BP elevation still exists. Decongestants are commonly found in combination or multi-ingredient cough and cold products. Inquire about their use, especially if the patient's BP has been well controlled at prior visits, then suddenly becomes elevated. If a decongestant is necessary, the nasal formulation can be considered, which has less systemic absorption.

Appetite suppressants or diet pills are another class of agents that can cause elevations in BP. Although weight loss may not be of primary concern in the elderly, these products usually contain a blend of various vitamins and herbal products as well as caffeine. Since no two products are manufactured the same, it is important to have the patient bring in the bottle(s), to review the ingredients and determine if this could be the cause of elevated BP.

NSAIDs are medications available by prescription or OTC. Of the most commonly used OTC products for those aged 65 years or older, ibuprofen and aspirin are among the top three.[24] These products can be used to treat a variety of conditions, but in the elderly population, the primary condition that comes to mind would be arthritic pain. These agents provide only symptomatic relief and do not alter the course of the disease progression.[25] The concern with NSAID use is that they cause salt and fluid retention, which can then lead to an increase in BP. If an elderly patient is looking for pain relief, acetaminophen may be considered as an alternative, which does not adversely affect BP.[26]

ADHERENCE/POLYPHARMACY

Medication nonadherence or polypharmacy can lead to an increase in hospital admissions and significant clinical and economic consequences, especially in the elderly. Medication adherence has been defined as the extent to which a patient's or caregiver's medication administration behavior coincides with medical advice. This term emphasizes effective communication between at least two people, the patient and the health care provider. It has been estimated that the true rate of medication adherence is about 50%.[27] In addition, one-half of all filled prescriptions in daily clinical practice are incorrectly taken.[28] Medication adherence is most likely to be achieved when there is an equal partnership between the patient and the health care team. Often the team will consist of many members, including the patient, primary care provider, nurse, pharmacist, caregivers, and family members. Even with all the support of others, very few patients are able to adhere to their prescribed medication regimen.[28] One study revealed that only one in six patients is able to maintain dosage intervals within the prescribed limits, adhere strictly to administration times, almost never miss a prescribed dose, and only occasionally take an extra dose.[29]

Medication nonadherence can lead to polypharmacy, and polypharmacy can also lead to nonadherence.[30] If a patient is nonadherent to his/her medications and this is unknown to the provider, additional agents may continually be added in an effort to control a patient's BP, leading to polypharmacy. With the population projected to live longer, there may be a valid indication for each and every medicine on the patient's medication profile. Data from the Slone survey had 44% of males using five or more medications, with the percentage for females being 57%. Polypharmacy increased from 54% to 67% during 5 years.[31] At least 90% of Americans older than 65 years take at least one medication daily, the majority take two or more medications, and two-thirds of the elderly in long-term care facilities receive three or more medications.[32] Because of the large number of medications patients may be taking (polypharmacy), some patients will become nonadherent to their regimens.

Various factors may affect medication adherence in the elderly. Balkrishnan[33] reviewed five factors as potential predictors of medication adherence in the elderly. The first category of factors influencing adherence is demographics. This includes age, race, sex, occupation, education level, and health literacy. It is important to assess if a patient is able to read and understand a prescription label along with the specific medication instructions. The second classification includes medical variables. Medical factors that may affect medication adherence include the type of diseases, severity and duration of the illness, number of comorbid conditions, frequent use of medical services, and patient satisfaction with health care providers. This can be especially important when considering a condition such as HTN in which many patients may not feel any symptoms, thus feeling no need to take their medication. A study by Morrell[34] showed that 3 months after starting treatment for HTN, about 50% of patients had discontinued treatment for HTN, whereas at 6 months, 50% to 60% of all treatments had been changed or discontinued. Other medical variables including patient's visual acuity, hearing, and manual dexterity all come into play when reading prescription bottle labels, opening the medication vials, and differentiating tablet color and appearance. Patients with medical conditions related to cognitive impairment, psychological stress, and depression are noted to have lower medication adherence rates. The third category of factors affecting medication adherence is the actual medication itself. The administration time, route of administration, type of medication, and adverse effects can determine whether a patient takes his/her medications as directed. Several antihypertensives are available in a once-daily dosing regimen and are preferred whenever possible. The number of concurrent medications a patient is taking may also influence adherence rates. The Seventh Report of the Joint National Committee on Prevention, Detection, Evaluation, and Treatment of High Blood Pressure noted that most patients would require two or more medications to control high BP.[35] This is in addition to the large number of medications the elderly may be taking for other chronic conditions. The fourth category relates to behavioral factors. This can include the provider-patient interactions and the patients' knowledge, understanding, and beliefs about their disease and medication. Patients who know and understand their health condition generally have better adherence, because they can perceive the need for treatment. Some patients may perceive their antihypertensive as not effective and "not making a difference." Another behavioral pattern that has been associated with nonadherence is patients taking a drug "holiday." This is when a patient intentionally takes time off from taking their medication. This can be very harmful, especially for medications such as antihypertensives, where nonadherence may precipitate a rebound effect, causing an increase in BP and heart rate. The opposite effect may also occur; if a patient has been off the antihypertensive medication for many days and then restarts at the same dose, he or she may precipitate the first-dose effect and experience postural hypotension. Another commonly observed behavior is improvement in medication adherence several days before a physician visit. Since obtaining serum drug concentrations is not a standard of care for antihypertensive medications, having patients track their home BP readings on a log may help a patient with adhering to regimens between office visits. The last classification of factors for medication adherence includes several economic variables. A patient's socioeconomic status, type of insurance coverage, out-of-pocket cost for medication and medical care, and income may affect adherence rates. Making sure that patients are on the preferred formulary agents from their insurance company can be 1 cost-saving strategy for the patient.[33] Many of the antihypertensive medications are now available in a generic version, making copayments for patients much less. Many nationwide chain pharmacies have reduced prices for certain generic medications.

Assessing Adherence

With medication adherence being a concern in the elderly, providers must have ways of assessing this in their patients. The Joint Commission on Accreditation of Healthcare Organizations (JCAHO) has defined *medication reconciliation* as the process of comparing a patient's medication orders to all of the medications that the patient has been taking.[36] This should be done to avoid medication errors, such as omissions, duplications, dosing errors, and drug interactions. Every office visit should include medication reconciliation. In most cases, it is not feasible to perform a pill count for every patient to assess the medication adherence rates. Instead, we rely on patient honesty through direct interview. It is important when asking patients about their medication not to use close-ended yes or no questions. By going through each medication in their chart and asking, "Please tell me how you take medication X," one can ascertain much more about their adherence. Patients often do not realize that they are taking a medication incorrectly until it is pointed out to them. By asking open-ended questions about medication regimens, one can also uncover any side effects or problems a patient may be experiencing with his/her medications. Visual problems may also impair the ability of an elderly patient from reading the directions accurately on the prescription bottle. Asking a patient to read the directions aloud can help discover this deficit. Prescription refill records may provide some evidence of adherence rates but is often difficult when patients get their medications filled from various pharmacies and have multiple physicians in different locations. Assessing a patient's medication adherence to the current regimen should be done before additional agents are considered for treatment.

The Prescribing Cascade

Often a medication is prescribed for a symptom that has not been recognized as being caused by another agent. By avoiding this prescribing cascade, the number of adverse drug reactions and polypharmacy can often be reduced. There are several instances when additional agents may be inappropriately added when managing or treating HTN. For example, a patient was recently started on a DHP calcium channel blocker for HTN. In 1 month, the patient presents with lower extremity edema and is started on a diuretic. In this case, rather than adding an additional agent for the edema, a better option would be switching the patient to a medication in a different class or decreasing the dose to determine if the edema resolves. Another example of the prescribing cascade would be a patient taking high doses of ibuprofen for osteoarthritis from a local drug store and presenting with a rise in BP, thus requiring an additional antihypertensive medication. A more reasonable choice for this patient would be to assess his or her need for NSAIDs and consider another agent without the adverse effects on BP. Another common example is a patient who may present with nocturia shortly after initiation of a diuretic for HTN. It is important to instruct patients to take the diuretic in the morning to prevent nocturia. Providers must always assess if presenting symptoms may be a result of prescription and/or nonprescription medications.

TRIALS/NECESSITY OF TREATMENT

With all the cautions and warnings associated with antihypertensive use in the elderly, the benefit of treating HTN in this population has been well documented in many trials. These include the Systolic Hypertension in the Elderly Program,[16] STOP-Hypertension,[18] Systolic Hypertension in Europe,[19] and Hypertension in the Very Elderly Trial;[17] these studies are reviewed in detail in another article in this journal.

The following recommendations should be considered when prescribing antihypertensive medications in the elderly to help decrease adverse reactions, prevent polypharmacy, and improve adherence.

GUIDELINES FOR PRESCRIBING ANTIHYPERTENSIVE MEDICATIONS TO ELDERLY PATIENTS

1. Take a thorough medication history including OTC, vitamin, and herbal products.
2. Screen for interactions: be aware of potential drug-drug, drug-disease, and drug-food interactions.
3. Estimate renal function: Glomerular–filtration rate should be measured or estimated in all patients and dose reductions should be taken if warranted.
4. "Start low and go slow:" Start with low doses as interindividual variability makes it impossible to predict the appropriate dose for every patient. Titrate the dose slowly and allow for longer than normal periods between dose adjustments to compensate for unpredictable interpatient pharmacodynamic and pharmacokinetic variability.
5. Simplify the therapeutic regimen whenever possible. Use combination medications when available to help improve adherence. Using once-daily medications can also increase adherence rates and lower pill burden.
6. Choose older medications. The older medications have more information available from studies in the elderly and can be used more predictably and reliably. The newer medications should only be considered if there is a clear advantage to their use in the elderly.
7. Suggest use of a pill box/medication organizer and/or reminder calendar.
8. Encourage use of the same pharmacy or pharmacy chain so that all prescription records are available and easily retrievable to screen for interactions and duplications in therapy.
9. Encourage the patient/caregiver to always carry a current list of medications including name, dose, and frequency.
10. Providers should be encouraged to write the indication for the medication in the directions, which will allow it to be included on the prescription label for the patient to view.

More chronic medical conditions often equate to more medications being used to treat those conditions. A study by Jyrrka and colleagues[31] described changes in medication use by an elderly cohort, 75 years and older, during a 5-year period. The investigators assessed medications taken regularly and on an as-needed basis, including vitamin usage. The average number of medications increased, from 6.3 to 7.5 medications, during a 5-year period. Overall, results showed that as the population aged, fewer as-needed medications were being used, whereas the number of regularly used medications increased. HTN is a perfect example of a chronic medical condition that requires scheduled medication treatment.

SUMMARY

Since the population is projected to be much older by mid century, treating chronic conditions such as HTN will become routine. Appropriate drug modifications must be made for the elderly to accommodate altered physiology, pharmacokinetics, and pharmacodynamics that accompany aging. The Beers criteria[13] is a tool developed to provide guidance with medication selection. HTN management in the elderly may require numerous agents, making medication consolidation important to reduce pill burden, out-of-pocket expense, as well as to avoid polypharmacy. Routine medication reconciliation should be done to assess adherence as well as screen for drug interactions. Encouraging patients to take an active role in their health care and understanding their medications and possible adverse effects can help improve adherence rates.

REFERENCES

1. Ogihara T, Hiwada K, Morimoto S, et al. Guidelines for treatment of hypertension in the elderly—2002 revised version. Hypertens Res 2003;26:1–36.
2. Elliott DP. Pharmacokinetics and pharmacodynamcies in the elderly. In: Schumock GT, Brundage DM, Chessman KH, et al, editors. Pharmacotherapy Self Assessment Program (5th Edition) Book 4: Geriatrics/Special Populations. Kansas City (MO): American College of Clinical Pharmacy; 2004. p. 115–30.
3. Williams L, Lowenthal DT. Drug therapy in the elderly. Southampt Med J 1992;85: 127–31.
4. Noble RE. Drug therapy in the elderly. Metabolism 2003;52:27–30.
5. Benet LZ, Kroetz DL, Sheiner LB. Pharmacokinetics: the dynamics of drug absorption, distribution, and elimination. In: Hardman JG, Limbird LE, editors. Goodman and Gilman's the pharmacological basis of therapeutics. 9th edition. New York: McGraw-Hill; 1996. p. 3–27.
6. Tanaka E. In vivo age-related changes in hepatic drug-oxidizing capacity in humans. J Clin Pharm Ther 1998;23:247–55.
7. Duthie EH Jr, Katz PR. Practice of Geriatrics. 3rd edition. Philadelphia: Saunders; 1998.
8. Bressler R, Bahl JJ. Principles of drug therapy for the elderly patient. Mayo Clin Proc 2003;78:1564–77.
9. McAinsh J, Holmes BF, Smith S, et al. Atenolol kinetics in renal failure. Clin Pharmacol Ther 1980;28:302–9.
10. AstraZeneca Pharmaceuticals, LP. Product information: TENORMIN(R). Wilmington (DE), AstraZeneca Pharmaceuticals, LP; 2005.
11. Vestal RE, Wood AJ, Shand DG. Reduced beta-adrenoceptor sensitivity in the elderly. Clin Pharmacol Ther 1979;26:181–6.
12. Goldberg RM, Mabee J, Chan L, et al. Drug-drug and drug-disease interactions in the ED: analysis of a high-risk population. Am J Emerg Med 1996;14:447–50.
13. Fick DM, Cooper JW, Wade WE, et al. Updating the Beers criteria for potentially inappropriate medication use in older adults: results of a US consensus panel of experts. Arch Intern Med 2003;163:2716–24.
14. Major cardiovascular events in hypertensive patients randomized to doxazosin vs chlorthalidone: the antihypertensive and lipid-lowering treatment to prevent heart attack trial (ALLHAT). ALLHAT Collaborative Research Group. JAMA 2000;283: 1967–75.
15. Pfizer, Inc. Product information: CARDURA(R). New York, Pfizer, Inc; 2008.
16. Prevention of stroke by antihypertensive drug treatment in older persons with isolated systolic hypertension. Final results of the Systolic Hypertension in the Elderly Program (SHEP). SHEP Cooperative Research Group. JAMA 1991;265: 3255–64.
17. Beckett NS, Peters R, Fletcher AE, et al. Treatment of hypertension in patients 80 years of age or older. N Engl J Med 2008;358:1887–98.

18. Dahlof B, Lindholm LH, Hansson L, et al. Morbidity and mortality in the Swedish Trial in Old Patients with Hypertension (STOP-Hypertension). Lancet 1991;338: 1281–5.
19. Staessen JA, Fagard R, Thijs L, et al. Randomised double-blind comparison of placebo and active treatment for older patients with isolated systolic hypertension. The Systolic Hypertension in Europe (Syst-Eur) Trial Investigators. Lancet 1997;350:757–64.
20. Wyeth Pharmaceuticals, Inc. Product information: INDERAL(R). Philadelphia (PA), Wyeth Pharmaceuticals, Inc; 2007.
21. Reserpine. Lexi Drugs Online, 2008. Lexi-Comp, Inc. Available at: http://online. lexi.com/crlsql/servlet/crlonline. Accessed September 28, 2008.
22. Spruill WT, WW. Diarrhea, constipation and irritable bowel syndrome. In: Dipiro JT, Talbert RC, Yee GC, et al, editors. Pharmacotherapy: a pathophysiological approach. 6th edition. New York: McGraw-Hill; 2005. p. 677–92.
23. Clonidine. Lexi Drugs Online,2008. Lexi-Comp, Inc. Available at: http://online.lexi. com/crlsql/servlet/crlonline. Accessed September 28, 2008.
24. Kaufman DW, Kelly JP, Rosenberg L, et al. Recent patterns of medication use in the ambulatory adult population of the United States: the Slone survey. JAMA 2002;287:337–44.
25. Chutka DS, Takahashi PY, Hoel RW. Inappropriate medications for elderly patients. Mayo Clin Proc 2004;79:122–39.
26. Hansen KE, Elliott ME. Osteoarthritis. In: Dipiro JT, Talbert RC, Yee GC, et al, editors. Pharmacotherapy: a pathophysiological approach. 6th edition. New York: McGraw-Hill; 2005. p. 1685–703.
27. Haynes RB, McDonald H, Garg AX, et al. Interventions for helping patients to follow prescriptions for medications. JAMA 2002;288:2868–79.
28. MacLaughlin EJ, Raehl CL, Treadway AK, et al. Assessing medication adherence in the elderly: which tools to use in clinical practice? Drugs Aging 2005;22: 231–55.
29. Urquhart J. Role of patient compliance in clinical pharmacokinetics. A review of recent research. Clin Pharm 1994;27:202–15.
30. Webster's Dictionary Online. Available at: http://www.websters-online-dictionary. org/definition/polypharmacy. Accessed September 28, 2008.
31. Jyrkka J, Vartiainen L, Hartikainen S, et al. Increasing use of medicines in elderly persons: a five-year follow-up of the Kuopio 75 + Study. Eur J Clin Pharmacol 2006;62:151–8.
32. Chutka DS, Evans JM, Fleming KC, et al. Symposium on geriatrics–Part I: drug prescribing for elderly patients. Mayo Clin Proc 1995;70:685–93.
33. Balkrishnan R. Predictors of medication adherence in the elderly. Clin Ther 1998; 20:764–71.
34. Morrell RW, Park DC, Kidder DP, et al. Adherence to antihypertensive medications across the life span. Gerontologist 1997;37:609–19.
35. Chobanian AV, Bakris GL, Black HR, et al. The Seventh Report of the Joint National Committee on Prevention, Detection, Evaluation, and Treatment of High Blood Pressure: the JNC 7 report. JAMA 2003;289:2560–72.
36. 2005 Joint Commission on Accreditation of Healthcare Organizations. 2005 hospitals' national patient safety goals. Oakbrook Terrace (IL): The Commission; 2005. Available at: http://www.jointcommission.org/SentinelEvents/SentinelEventAlert/ sea_35.htm. Accessed September 28, 2008.
37. Onusko E. Diagnosing secondary hypertension. Am Fam Physician 2003;67: 67–74.

Drug Treatment of Hypertension in Older Hypertensives

Arash Rashidi, MD[a], Jackson T. Wright, Jr, MD, PhD[a,b],*

KEYWORDS

- Hypertension • Treatment • Elderly
- Antihypertensives • Geriatrics

The overriding goal of treatment of hypertension is to prevent its complications. This is particularly important in populations such as the elderly, the population at highest risk for complications (see the article by Mosley and Lloyd-Jones, elsewhere in this issue). Since the ability to assess the effect of antihypertensive treatment is not evident until years after it is started, it is critical that treatment selection is based on the best evidence that the treatment selected will address the primary reason for treating the disorder, the reduction of hypertension morbidity and mortality. We now have very strong evidence supporting the benefit of antihypertensive treatment in older patients and data to assess treatment with most classes of antihypertensive agents. Most of the studies demonstrating the benefit of antihypertensive drug therapy were, in fact, conducted in patients 55 years of age and older (**Table 1**). The objective of this issue is to review the evidence base for the recommendations for antihypertensive drug therapy in the older hypertensive patient.

EVIDENCE BASE FOR HYPERTENSION TREATMENT IN THE ELDERLY
Blood Pressure Lowering

Summary data from trials designed to evaluate the effect of treating to different blood pressure (BP) goals are shown at the top of **Table 1**. Early hypertension morbidity and mortality trials focused on treating to diastolic blood pressure (DBP) goals.[1–3] In the early 1990s, trials directed at evaluating the effect of lowering systolic blood pressure (SBP) began to be reported.[4–6] These latter trials were invariably conducted in older patients and documented substantial lowering of cardiovascular (CV) morbidity and mortality with SBP lowering.

[a] Department of Medicine, Case Western Reserve University, 29325 Health Campus Drive, Suit#3, Westlake, Ohio 44145, USA
[b] Clinical Hypertension Program, William T Dahms Clinical Research Unit, Bolwell Suite 2200, 11100 Euclid Avenue, Cleveland, OH 44106-6053, USA
* Clinical Hypertension Program, William T Dahms Clinical Research Unit, Bolwell Suite 2200, 11100 Euclid Avenue, Cleveland, OH 44106-6053.
E-mail address: jackson.wright@case.edu (J. Wright).

Clin Geriatr Med 25 (2009) 235–244
doi:10.1016/j.cger.2009.03.001
0749-0690/09/$ – see front matter © 2009 Elsevier Inc. All rights reserved.

geriatric.theclinics.com

Table 1
Antihypertensive treatment clinical outcome trials

Trial	Intervention	Age (y)	Stroke	MI	HF	All CVD	Mortality	ESRD
			Outcome (% reduction, *P*)					
Antihypertensive treatment vs placebo (PLCB) or Usual Care (UC)								
VA-COOP[1]	THZD-based vs PLCB	52	—	—	—	—	—	—
HDFP[2]	THZD-based vs UC	51	—	—	—	—	17[b]	—
EWPHE[3]	THZD-based vs PLCB	72 ± 8	ns	ns	—	36[b]	ns	ns
SHEP[4]	THZD-based vs PLCB	71 ± 7	—	—	—	—	—	—
Sys-Eur[6]	CCB-based vs PLCB	70 ± 7	44[b]	ns	ns	31[b]	ns	ns
Sys-China[5]	CCB vs PLCB	67 ± 6	38[b]	ns	ns	37[b]	39[b]	ns
HYVET[42]	THZD-ACEI vs PLCB	84 ± 3	30 ns	ns	64[b]	34[b]	21[a]	—
HOPE[43]	ACEI vs UC-PLCB	66 ÷ 7	32[b]	20[b]	23[b]	22[b]	16[b]	—
PROGRESS[37]	ACEI-THZD vs UC-PLCB	64 ± 10	28[b]	ns	—	26[b]	ns	—
ACE Inhibitor/ARB comparison								
CAPPP[44]	ACEI vs THZD-BB	56 ± 8	−25[a]	ns	ns	ns	ns	—
LIFE[45]	ARB vs BB	67 ± 7	25[b]	ns	ns	13[b]	ns	ns
VALUE[38]	ARB vs DHP-CCB	67 ± 8	ns	−19[a]	ns	ns	ns	ns
ONTARGET[52]	ACEI vs ARB	66 ± 7	ns	ns	ns	ns	ns	ns
	ACEI vs ARB +ACEI	66 ± 7	ns	ns	ns	ns	ns	ns
Calcium Channel Blocker (CCB) comparisons								
NORDIL[46]	CCB vs THZD-BB	60 ± 7	20[a]	ns	—	ns	ns	—
ASCOT[47]	DHP-CCB vs BB	63 ± 9	23[b]	13[a]	ns	16[b]	11[a]	—
INSIGHT[24]	DHP-CCB vs THZD	65 ± 7	ns	ns	55[a]	ns	ns	ns
CONVINCE[48]	CCB vs THZD-BB	66 ± 7	ns	ns	30[a]	ns	ns	ns
Beta Blocker (BB) comparisons								
MRC in Elderly[49]	BB vs THZD	70	ns	−40[b]	—	−29[b]	19 ns	—
LIFE[45]	BB vs ARB	67 ± 7	−25[b]	ns	ns	−13[b]	ns	ns
ASCOT[47]	BB vs DHP-CCB	63 ± 9	−23[b]	−13[a]	ns	−16[b]	−11[a]	—
Diuretic (THZD) comparisons								
ALLHAT[32]	THZD vs α-blocker	67 ± 8	26[b]	ns	80[b]	20[b]	ns	ns
ALLHAT[31,40]	THZD vs DHP-CCB	67 ± 8	ns	ns	38[b]	ns	ns	ns
ALLHAT[31,40]	THZD vs ACEI	67 ± 8	15[a]	ns	19[b]	10[b]	ns	ns
ACCOMPLISH[36]	THZD-ACEI vs CCB-ACEI	68 ± 7	ns	−22[a]	ns	−20[b]	ns	ns

Abbreviations: DHP-CCB, dihydropyridine calcium channel blocker; ns, not statistically significant; PLCB, placebo; THZD, thiazide diuretic; *UC*, usual care.
[a] $P<0.05$.
[b] $P<0.01$.

There remains uncertainty regarding the appropriate BP goal in older hypertensive patients. Although there is now consensus on a BP goal of less than 140/90 mm Hg even in older patients, some recent guidelines recommend even lower goals, especially in high-risk patients.[7,8] Observational data suggest that risk of hypertensive complications decrease down to SBP levels as low 115 mm Hg with increasing absolute risk of vascular and total mortality with each decade of age.[7,9] In addition, post hoc analyses of a number of clinical outcome trials that involved older patients also suggest better outcomes when lower SBPs are achieved even in study cohorts where all SBPs are less than 140 mm Hg (**Table 2**) Furthermore, in meta-analyses of different treatment regimens, with the exception of heart failure (HF), differences in CV outcomes were largely accounted for by differences in achieved BP.[10,11] These findings appear to support a BP goal less than the currently recommended less than 140/90 mm Hg. However, the SBP differences between treatment arms have been small in these trials, and the lack of randomization makes interpretation of the differences in outcome relative to the BP differences difficult. Thus, it is unclear whether the benefit is due to the difference in achieved BP or unaccounted for differences in disease risk unrelated to BP. Finally, albeit the concerns about the data raised in the article by Mosley and Lloyd-Jones, elsewhere in this issue, the analyses suggesting increased coronary heart disease (CHD) risk with DBP lowering below 60 mm Hg leave room for caution.[12–15]

Thus, clinical trial evidence of benefit for SBP levels that approach the current goal of less than 140/90 mm Hg is strong, but a definitive trial of lowering SBP to a goal substantially less than 140 mm Hg SBP is not yet available. The Action to Control Cardiovascular Risk in Diabetes trial is currently evaluating the effect of an SBP goal less than 120 mm Hg compared with one less than 140 mm Hg in a diabetic cohort.[16,17] With a mean baseline BP of 135/75 mm Hg (and mean pulse pressure, 60 mm Hg) in a cohort obviously at high risk for CHD, it should provide valuable information on this topic.[17] A similar trial sponsored by National Institutes of Health in nondiabetics is planned to begin in 2011.

EVIDENCE SUPPORTING ANTIHYPERTENSIVE DRUG SELECTION IN THE OLDER PATIENT
Blood Pressure-Lowering Efficacy in the Older Patient

Earlier studies suggested increasing resistance with age to the BP-lowering effects of drugs acting on the renin-angiotensin system (RAS) (ie, beta blockers, angiotensin-converting enzyme inhibitors [ACEI], angiotensin receptor blockers [ARBs]) compared with calcium channel blockers (CCBs) and thiazide diuretics (THZD).[18,19] This was suggested to be related to the reduction in plasma renin activity with age. Recent studies show substantial heterogeneity of response, with these agents making age less of a predictor of response and similar BP lowering across antihypertensive classes (**Table 3**).[20] However, less BP-lowering efficacy is seen with these agents in black hypertensive patients regardless of age.[21]

Table 2
Difference in achieved blood pressure and effect on clinical outcomes

Trial	HOPE[43]	EUROPA[50]	PROGRESS[37]	CAMELOT[51]	ALLHAT-THZ vs ACEI[31]	ALLHAT-THZ vs CCB[31]	ALLHAT-THZ vs α-B[32]
Achieved BP	139/77 vs 136/76	133/80 vs. 128/78	—	~130/78	136/75 vs. 134/75	135/75 vs. 134/75	140/80 vs 137/79
Δ BP	3/1	5/2	9/4	5/2	2/0	1/−1	3/1
Outcome (% ↓)							
Stroke	32	—	28	—	15	−7	26
CHD	22	20	38	—	5	0	−3
HF	23	39	n/a	—	38	19	80
All CVD	22	14	26	31[a]	10	4	20
ESRD	—	—	—	—	11	12	−4

[a] Mostly hospitalized angina and revascularization with amlodipine.

Table 3 Reduction in SBP by antihypertensive medications by age and race[20]				
	Whites ≤60 y Old (N=243)	Blacks ≤60 y Old (N=288)	Whites >60 y Old (N=405)	Blacks >60 y Old (N=330)
Placebo	5 ± 10 mm Hg	0.5 ± 10 mm Hg	3 ± 10 mm Hg	3 ± 11 mm Hg
Captopril (25–50 mg BID)	11 ± 9 mm Hg	8 ± 11 mm Hg	11 ± 9 mm Hg	7 ± 12 mm Hg
Atenolol (25–100 mg/d)	14 ± 11 mm Hg	7 ± 11 mm Hg	12 ± 14 mm Hg	9 ± 11 mm Hg
Diltiazem (60–180 mg BID)	11 ± 9 mm Hg	14 ± 10 mm Hg	12 ± 9 mm Hg	15 ± 7 mm Hg
HCTZ (12.5–50 mg/d)	12 ± 11 mm Hg	14 ± 9 mm Hg	13 ± 12 mm Hg	16 ± 11 mm Hg
Prazosin (2–10 mg BID)	8 ± 9 mm Hg	8 ± 12 mm Hg	17 ± 12 mm Hg	13 ± 13 mm Hg
Clonidine (0.1–0.3 mg BID)	16 ± 12 mm Hg	13 ± 10 mm Hg	17 ± 13 mm Hg	17 ± 15 mm Hg

Evidence on the Effectiveness of Drug Classes in Preventing Clinical Outcomes

Reduction in CV events with BP lowering was first documented in placebo-controlled trials, initially with diuretic and beta blocker-based therapy and subsequently with ACEI and CCBs (see **Table 1**). Even in these studies, mean age was at least more than 50 years. In the 1990s, after the initial trials demonstrating the benefit of BP lowering, the focus of investigation shifted to differentiating the relative benefit of the various antihypertensive regimens.[10] These trials generally studied older patients (with diabetics or other high-risk groups) to exploit the higher event rate permitting a smaller sample size.

Evidence with Calcium Channel Blockers

The effectiveness of CCBs in preventing hypertensive complications was first demonstrated in an elderly cohort with isolated systolic hypertension (ISH).[22] This was followed by the STOP-Hypertension-2 trial in 6,614 severely hypertensive patients between age 70 to 84 years, with an SBP greater than or equal to 180 mm Hg and/ or a DBP greater than or equal to 105 mm Hg.[23] Participants in this study were randomized to either a dihydropyridine CCB (felodipine or isradipine) or an ACEI (enalapril or lisinopril), both compared with conventional therapy with a beta blocker or THZD. No differences were seen between treatment arms in rates of CV mortality or major events, although the study had limited power to detect less than dramatic (>25%) differences between regimens. The Intervention as a Goal in Hypertension Treatment trial compared sustained-release Nifedipine 30 to 60 mg/d to Hydrochlorothiazide (HCTZ) (25–50 mg/d)/amiloride 2.5 to 5 mg/d.[24] No difference in the primary composite CVD outcome was noted, but a doubling in risk of HF was noted (relative risk, 2.2; CI, 1.07–4.49; P=.028). This pattern of similar BP reduction, overall CVD incidence, but lesser protection against HF compared with THZDs was also seen in the Antihypertensive and Lipid-Lowering to Prevent Heart Attack Trial (ALLHAT) (see the following sections) and trials with the CCBs diltiazem (NORDIL) and verapamil (CONVINCE) (see **Table 1**).

Evidence with Renin-Angiotensin System Inhibitors

The renin-angiotensin system inhibitors (RASI) were initially evaluated in diabetic patients. The studies most relevant to older hypertensive patients began with the United Kingdom Prospective Diabetes Study, which found no difference in outcomes between an ACEI and beta blocker regimen on diabetic outcomes although under-powered (n = 1148) for CVD (see **Table 1**). This was followed by the Captopril Prevention Project (CAPPP), a large (n = 10,985), open-label trial, which compared the effects of antihypertensive treatment initiated with an ACEI versus THZD/beta blocker-based therapy on CV morbidity and mortality in a predominantly nondiabetic population. No difference was seen in the rate of fatal and nonfatal myocardial infarction and CV mortality, but stroke was 25% more common with captopril (P = .04). A diabetic subgroup in this study randomized to the ACEI did have a lower rate of CV events, including coronary events and CV mortality. The Heart Outcomes Prevention Evaluation (HOPE) trial (n = 9297) compared an ACEI versus placebo in an older cohort of hypertensive and nonhypertensive participants with or at high risk for CVD and reported dramatic differences in CVD outcomes (see **Table 1**). The ARBs have also shown effectiveness in preventing hypertension outcomes in CVD and renal outcome trials but are no better in preventing outcomes than ACEI and have little additive benefit in combination with ACEI (see **Table 1**).[25] They are better tolerated than ACEI, that is, less likely to cause cough or angioedema. Direct renin inhibitors have been released in 2007 but to date have shown no advantage over ACEI or ARBs.[26] RAS inhibitors are less effective in lowering BP and in preventing complications in black hypertensive patients unless combined with diuretics or CCBs (see the following subsections). Older black hypertensive patients are also more likely to experience cough and angioedema with ACEI.[21,27]

Evidence with Beta Blockers

The beta blockers have recently undergone reevaluation in light of newer data.[28–30] Although earlier studies showed them to be effective in preventing clinical outcomes against placebo, they have been shown less CVD protection in large comparative outcome trials against diuretics, CCBs, and ARBs (see **Table 1**). Thus, for CVD primary prevention in older hypertensive patients without CHD or HF, beta blockers should be considered second-line agents along with alpha blockers and other sympatholytics.

Evidence with Diuretics

Most of the early data showing benefit of antihypertensive therapy in preventing hypertension morbidity and mortality were those obtained in trials conducted using THZD (see **Table 1**). In comparative trials with other classes of antihypertensives, THZD have remained unsurpassed in preventing hypertensive complications, particularly in the elderly. The largest of these, ALLHAT confirmed the findings of other studies that neither an ACEI, CCB, or alpha-blocker-initiated therapy surpassed therapy initiated with a THZD in lowering BP or in preventing CVD or renal outcomes.[27,31–33] Overall, THZD-based therapy was superior to alpha blocker, ACEI, and CCB-based therapies in preventing 1 or more major forms of CVD, including stroke and HF. It was superior to alpha-blocker-based therapy in preventing overall CVD, especially HF and stroke, and superior to the ACEI-based regimen in preventing overall CVD, including stroke (in black persons only), HF, angina, and coronary revascularizations. Compared with CCB-based therapy, THZD-based therapy was similar in overall CVD protection but superior in preventing HF. These results in ALLHAT were consistent by age, sex, diabetic status, and level of renal function for all outcomes, and by race, except for stroke and overall CVD.[27] Neither the CCB-based nor the ACEI-based regimens were superior to the THZD-based regimen in preventing end-stage renal disease overall or when stratified by diabetes or baseline estimated glomerular filtration rate.[33,34] These results are also confirmed by two major meta-analyses.[10,35]

In ALLHAT, as in other studies, a 5 mg/dL increase in glucose was noted in the THZD arm compared with those on the ACEI. This resulted in a significantly greater number of participants crossing the 126-mg/dL threshold defining diabetes. Despite the data showing that diuretics were at least as effective as the other treatment arms in preventing major clinical outcomes, the focus was changed from the small absolute increase in glucose levels to the long-term significance of "diuretic-associated, new-onset diabetes." Reanalysis of the ALLHAT data and other studies have since shown that as much as a 10-mg/dL increase in glucose during the trial resulted in no subsequent significant increase in CVD.[27] Importantly, the increase in aggregate clinical CVD associated with both incident diabetes and a 10-mg/dL increase in glucose was lowest in the chlorthalidone arm and highest in the lisinopril arm, with the CCB arm intermediate or similar.

Only two studies appear to challenge the findings in ALLHAT and other studies. An Australian study (Australian National Blood Pressure Study [ANBP2]) in a very small cohort compared a THZD-based regiment to one containing an ACEI and found a significant benefit of the ACEI on CVD outcomes in men only. It had approximately 1/4 the participants (6083 versus 24,309 in ALLHAT for THZD and ACEI arms) and 1/5 to 1/10 the CVD endpoints as ALLHAT. It also had an open-label design, and only 83% of subjects in ANBP2 ever received assigned treatment, and only 58% of subjects randomly assigned to ACEI and 62% of those assigned to diuretic were still receiving assigned treatment at the end of the study (83% and 89% in ALLHAT). More recently, the Avoiding Cardiovascular events through COMBination therapy in Patients LIving with Systolic Hypertension (ACCOMPLISH) trial evaluated two fixed combinations, one consisting of an ACEI (benazepril) and a CCB (amlodipine) compared with one containing the same dose of benazepril and a THZD (HCTZ).[36] This trial was stopped by its Data Safety and Monitoring Board when the difference in the primary endpoint between the two arms crossed the prespecified boundary favoring the CCB/ACEI combination (risk ratio, 0.81; $P = .0002$). It is worth noting that the treatment arms contained the same dose of benazepril (40 mg/d) in the two arms and the dose of amlodipine (5–10 mg/d) that was used in previous outcome trials. However, the HCTZ dose (12.5–25 mg/d) was only half the dose (HCTZ 25–50 mg/d or 12.5–25 mg/d of the more potent chlorthalidone) used in trials showing benefit of THZD in preventing CVD outcomes. Thus, the ACCOMPLISH trial reminds us that providers should use drug doses shown to be effective in clinical outcome trials. The ACCOMPLISH trial suggests that HCTZ at 12.5 to 25 mg/d cannot be recommended. HCTZ should be titrated to 25 to 50 mg/d. Outcome data support chlorthalidone at 12.5 to 25 mg/d and indapamide at 2.5 mg/d.[37]

PRINCIPLES OF TREATING THE OLDER HYPERTENSIVE PATIENT

Particularly in the older hypertensive patient, aggressive efforts to assist with lifestyle changes should be incorporated into his or her regimen. BP goal and drug selection in the elderly are similar to those in younger populations, but there are a few special considerations in these patients. First, the focus of treatment should be on achieving an SBP goal of less than 140 mm Hg. Achieving the DBP goal in older hypertensive patients is comparatively easy; the SBP goal is the more challenging. Secondly, the clinical trial data indicate that unlike in younger hypertensive patients, the benefits of treatment in preventing major CV morbidity and mortality can be appreciated within 2 to 5 years. Thus, it is unfortunate that hypertensive patients older than age 65 years continue to have the lowest rates of achieving goal BPs. Medication can be started with lower doses than those for younger patients, and BP reduction should be more gradual. However, it is critical to avoid the commonly observed clinical inertia, and some studies have suggested an increase in CVD events with delayed BP reduction.[38,39] Finally, because of the high prevalence of orthostatic hypotension in the older hypertensive patient, standing BPs should be routinely measured, and treatment may be influenced by the standing values.

The evidence outlined here and meta-analyses of clinical outcome trials during the past decade have shown that although differences in specific outcomes and in selected populations may be evident, the differences between drug regimens on overall CV outcomes are relatively small compared with the differences between different BP levels.[10,31,32,40] In addition, it is now clear that most hypertensive patients will require multiple agents to reach their BP goal. Seventh Report of the Joint National Committee on Prevention, Detection, Evaluation and Treatment of High Blood Pressure promoted thiazide-type diuretics as initial therapy in most hypertensive patients because of their overall utility in lowering BP, their synergistic or additive effect in combination with other agents in lowering BP, and their lower cost, in addition to the fact that no other class surpassed them in preventing hypertensive complications. However, since it is likely that combinations of these and other classes of antihypertensive agents will be required to achieve the BP goals, their implications on the trial design will likely be minimal.

The best evidence and most guidelines still recommend the inclusion of a THZD as one of the agents in the regimen. An additional advantage of THZD in older patients is their tendency for a positive calcium balance and decrease in the risk of fracture.[41] The long-acting THZDs (chlorthalidone or metolazone) may be considered in those who experience urgency with shorter-acting agents such as HCTZ. CCBs remain an excellent alternative in those unable to take a THZD, especially in black patients. In those without a specific indication for their use (HF, chronic kidney disease) RASIs are excellent additions to the regimen. Beta blocker use in older hypertensives should be reserved for additional BP lowering in those not controlled on a diuretic, dihydropyridine CCB, and RASI or if there are specific indications, for example, post MI, angina or HF. In resistant hypertensives, evaluation for secondary causes should be undertaken. Spironolactone or eplerenone is often effective in resistant hypertensive patients and can be added even in those without hyperaldosteronism.

REFERENCES

1. Effects of treatment on morbidity in hypertension. II. Results in patients with diastolic blood pressure averaging 90 through 114 mm Hg. JAMA 1970;213(7): 1143–52.
2. Five-year findings of the hypertension detection and follow-up program. I. Reduction in mortality of persons with high blood pressure, including mild hypertension. Hypertension Detection and Follow-up Program Cooperative Group. JAMA 1979; 242(23):2562–71.
3. Amery A, Birkenhager W, Brixko P, et al. Mortality and morbidity results from the European Working Party on High Blood Pressure in the Elderly trial. Lancet 1985; 325(8442):1349–54.
4. Prevention of stroke by antihypertensive drug treatment in older persons with isolated systolic hypertension. Final results of the Systolic Hypertension in the Elderly Program (SHEP). SHEP Cooperative Research Group. JAMA 1991;265(24):3255–64.
5. Liu L, Wang JG, Gong L, et al. Comparison of active treatment and placebo in older Chinese patients with isolated systolic hypertension. Systolic Hypertension in China (Syst-China) Collaborative Group. J Hypertens 1998;16(12 Pt 1):1823–9.

6. Staessen JA, Fagard R, Thijs L, et al. Randomised double-blind comparison of placebo and active treatment for older patients with isolated systolic hypertension. The Systolic Hypertension in Europe (Syst-Eur) Trial Investigators. Lancet 1997;350(9080):757–64.

7. Chobanian AV, Bakris GL, Black HR, et al. The Seventh Report of the Joint National Committee on prevention, detection, evaluation, and treatment of high blood pressure: the JNC 7 report. JAMA 2003;289(19):2560–72.

8. Fraker TD Jr, Fihn SD, Gibbons RJ, et al. 2007 chronic angina focused update of the ACC/AHA 2002 Guidelines for the management of patients with chronic stable angina: a report of the American College of Cardiology/American Heart Association Task Force on Practice Guidelines Writing Group to develop the focused update of the 2002 Guidelines for the management of patients with chronic stable angina. Circulation 2007;116(23):2762–72.

9. Lewington S, Clarke R, Qizilbash N, et al. Age-specific relevance of usual blood pressure to vascular mortality: a meta-analysis of individual data for one million adults in 61 prospective studies. Lancet 2002;360(9349):1903–13.

10. Turnbull F. Effects of different blood-pressure-lowering regimens on major cardiovascular events: results of prospectively-designed overviews of randomised trials. Lancet 2003;362(9395):1527–35.

11. Staessen JA, Wang JG, Thijs L. Cardiovascular protection and blood pressure reduction: a meta-analysis. Lancet 2001;358(9290):1305–15.

12. Hansson L. The J-shaped curve. In: Laragh JH, Brenner BM, editors. Hypertension: pathophysiology, diagnosis, and management. New York: Raven Press; 1995. p. 2765–70.

13. Somes GW, Pahor M, Shorr RI, et al. The role of diastolic blood pressure when treating isolated systolic hypertension. Arch Intern Med 1999;159(17):2004–9.

14. Messerli FH, Mancia G, Conti CR, et al. Dogma disputed: can aggressively lowering blood pressure in hypertensive patients with coronary artery disease be dangerous? Ann Intern Med 2006;144(12):884–93.

15. Fagard RH, Staessen JA, Thijs L, et al. On-treatment diastolic blood pressure and prognosis in systolic hypertension. Arch Intern Med 2007;167(17):1884–91.

16. Buse JB, Bigger JT, Byington RP, et al. Action to Control Cardiovascular Risk in Diabetes (ACCORD) trial: design and methods. Am J Cardiol 2007;99(12A):21i–33i.

17. Gerstein HC, Miller ME, Byington RP, et al. Effects of intensive glucose lowering in type 2 diabetes. N Engl J Med 2008;358(24):2545–59.

18. Buhler FR. Antihypertensive treatment according to age, plasma renin and race. Drugs 1988;35:495–503.

19. Williams GH. Converting-enzyme inhibitors in the treatment of hypertension. N Engl J Med 1988;319(23):1517–25.

20. Materson BJ, Reda DJ, Cushman WC, et al. Single-drug therapy for hypertension in men. A comparison of six antihypertensive agents with placebo. The Department of Veterans Affairs Cooperative Study Group on Antihypertensive Agents. N Engl J Med 1993;328(13):914–21.

21. Johnson EF, Wright JT Jr. Management of hypertension in Black populations. In: Oparil S, Weber M, editors. Hypertension. A companion to Brenner and Rector's: the kidney. Philadelphia: Elsevier; 2005. p. 587–602.

22. Gasowski J, Birkenhager WH, Staessen JA, et al. Benefit of antihypertensive treatment in the diabetic patients enrolled in the Systolic Hypertension in Europe (Syst-Eur) trial. Cardiovasc Drugs Ther 2000;14(1):49–53.

23. Hansson L, Lindholm LH, Ekbom T, et al. Randomised trial of old and new antihypertensive drugs in elderly patients: cardiovascular mortality and morbidity the

Swedish Trial in Old Patients with Hypertension-2 study. Lancet 1999;354(9192): 1751–6.

24. Brown MJ, Palmer CR, Castaigne A, et al. Morbidity and mortality in patients randomised to double-blind treatment with a long-acting calcium-channel blocker or diuretic in the International Nifedipine GITS study: Intervention as a Goal in Hypertension Treatment (INSIGHT). Lancet 2000;356(9227):366–72.

25. Yusuf S, Teo KK, Pogue J, et al. Telmisartan, ramipril, or both in patients at high risk for vascular events. N Engl J Med 2008;358(15):1547–59.

26. Oparil S, Yarows SA, Patel S, et al. Dual inhibition of the renin system by aliskiren and valsartan. Lancet 2007;370(9593):1126–7

27. Wright JTJr, Probsltield J, Cushman WC, et al. ALLHAT findings revisited in the context of subsequent analyses, other trials, and meta-analyses. Arch Intern Med 2009;169(9):1–11.

28. Messerli FH, Grossman E, Goldbourt U. Are beta-blockers efficacious as first-line therapy for hypertension in the elderly? A systematic review. JAMA 1998;279(23): 1903–7.

29. Lindholm LH, Carlberg B, Samuelsson O. Should beta blockers remain first choice in the treatment of primary hypertension? A meta-analysis. Lancet 2005; 366(9496):1545–53.

30. National Collaborating Centre for Chronic Conditions. Hypertension: management of hypertension in adults in primary care: partial update. London: Royal College of Physicians; 2006.

31. Antihypertensive and Lipid-Lowering Treatment to Prevent Heart Attack Trial Collaborative Research Group. The ALLHAT Officers and Coordinators for the ALLHAT Collaborative Research Group. Major outcomes in high-risk hypertensive patients randomized to angiotensin-converting enzyme inhibitor or calcium channel blocker vs diuretic: The Antihypertensive and Lipid-Lowering Treatment to Prevent Heart Attack Trial (ALLHAT). JAMA 2002;288(23):2981–97.

32. Diuretic versus alpha-blocker as first-step antihypertensive therapy: final results from the Antihypertensive and Lipid-Lowering Treatment to Prevent Heart Attack Trial (ALLHAT). Hypertension 2003;42(3):239–46.

33. Rahman M, Pressel S, Davis BR, et al. Renal outcomes in high-risk hypertensive patients treated with an angiotensin-converting enzyme inhibitor or a calcium channel blocker vs a diuretic: a report from the Antihypertensive and Lipid-Lowering Treatment to Prevent Heart Attack Trial (ALLHAT). Arch Intern Med 2005;165(8):936–46.

34. Wright JT Jr, Harris-Haywood S, Pressel S, et al. Clinical outcomes by race in hypertensive patients with and without the metabolic syndrome in ALLHAT. Arch Intern Med 2008;168:1–11.

35. Psaty BM, Smith NL, Siscovick DS, et al. Health outcomes associated with antihypertensive therapies used as first-line agents. A systematic review and meta-analysis. JAMA 1997;277(9):739–45.

36. Jamerson K, Weber MA, Bakris GL, et al. Benazepril plus amlodipine or hydrochlorothiazide for hypertension in high-risk patients. N Engl J Med 2008; 359(23):2417–28.

37. PROGRESS Collaborative Group. Randomised trial of a perindopril-based blood-pressure-lowering regimen among 6,105 individuals with previous stroke or transient ischaemic attack. Lancet 2001;358(9287):1033–41.

38. Julius S, Kjeldsen SE, Weber M, et al. Outcomes in hypertensive patients at high cardiovascular risk treated with regimens based on valsartan or amlodipine: the VALUE randomised trial. Lancet 2004;363(9426):2022–31.

39. Weber MA, Julius S, Kjeldsen SE, et al. Blood pressure dependent and independent effects of antihypertensive treatment on clinical events in the VALUE Trial. Lancet 2004;363(9426):2049–51.
40. Wright JT Jr, Dunn JK, Cutler JA, et al. Outcomes in hypertensive black and nonblack patients treated with chlorthalidone, amlodipine, and lisinopril. JAMA 2005;293(13):1595–608.
41. Jones G, Nguyen T, Sambrook PN, et al. Thiazide diuretics and fractures: can meta-analysis help? J Bone Miner Res 1995;10(1):106–11.
42. Beckett NS, Peters R, Fletcher AE, et al. Treatment of hypertension in patients 80 years of age or older. N Engl J Med 2008;358(18):1887–98.
43. Yusuf S, Sleight P, Pogue J, et al. Effects of an angiotensin-converting-enzyme inhibitor, ramipril, on cardiovascular events in high-risk patients. The Heart Outcomes Prevention Evaluation Study Investigators. N Engl J Med 2000; 342(3):145–53.
44. Hansson L, Lindholm LH, Niskanen L, et al. Effect of angiotensin-converting-enzyme inhibition compared with conventional therapy on cardiovascular morbidity and mortality in hypertension: the Captopril Prevention Project (CAPPP) randomised trial. Lancet 1999;353(9153):611–6.
45. Dahlof B, Devereux RB, Kjeldsen SE, et al. Cardiovascular morbidity and mortality in the Losartan Intervention For Endpoint reduction in hypertension study (LIFE): a randomised trial against atenolol. Lancet 2002;359(9311): 995–1003.
46. Hansson L, Hedner T, Lund-Johansen P, et al. Randomised trial of effects of calcium antagonists compared with diuretics and beta-blockers on cardiovascular morbidity and mortality in hypertension: the Nordic Diltiazem (NORDIL) study. Lancet 2000;356(9227):359–65.
47. Dahlof B, Sever PS, Poulter NR, et al. Prevention of cardiovascular events with an antihypertensive regimen of amlodipine adding perindopril as required versus atenolol adding bendroflumethiazide as required, in the Anglo-Scandinavian Cardiac Outcomes Trial-Blood Pressure Lowering Arm (ASCOT-BPLA): a multicentre randomised controlled trial. Lancet 2005;366(9489):895–906.
48. Black HR, Elliott WJ, Grandits G, et al. Principal results of the Controlled Onset Verapamil Investigation of Cardiovascular End Points (CONVINCE) trial. JAMA 2003;289(16):2073–82.
49. Medical Research Council trial of treatment of hypertension in older adults: principal results. MRC Working Party. BMJ 1992;304(6824):405–12.
50. Fox KM. Efficacy of perindopril in reduction of cardiovascular events among patients with stable coronary artery disease: randomised, double-blind, placebo-controlled, multicentre trial (the EUROPA study). Lancet 2003; 362(9386):782–8.
51. Nissen SE, Tuzcu EM, Libby P, et al. Effect of antihypertensive agents on cardiovascular events in patients with coronary disease and normal blood pressure: the CAMELOT study: a randomized controlled trial. JAMA 2004;292(18):2217–25.
52. The ONTARGET Investigator. Telmisartan, Ramipril, or Both in Patients at High Risk for Vascular Events. NEJM 2008;358:1547–9.

Renin Angiotensin System Inhibition in the Older Person: A Review

Maha A. Mohamed, MD, Matthew R. Weir, MD*

KEYWORDS

• Renin angiotensin system • Hypertension • Cardiovascular
• Kidney • RAS blocking • Older persons

The efficacy and safety of renin angiotensin system (RAS) inhibition for lowering blood pressure in older populations has been demonstrated in a number of clinical trials. Whether a patient's age influences the overall ability of these drugs to lower blood pressure and protect against progress of cardiovascular and kidney disease has been the focus of few clinical trials. Herein, we review the mechanism of action of the renin angiotensin cascade and then discuss the clinical evidence surrounding the use of RAS-blocking drugs in the older population.

RENIN ANGIOTENSIN SYSTEM BLOCKADE

RAS is an autocrine, paracrine, and enzymatic cascade that can regulate blood pressure, cell proliferation, and vascular remodeling.[1] Renin is synthesized by the juxtaglomerular cells in the afferent glomerular arterioles in the kidney. The release of renin occurs in response to certain physiologic stimuli, such as renal hypoperfusion, that occur in the setting of volume depletion and hypotension.

Renin release leads to cleavage of angiotensin I from angiotensinogen, which is primarily produced in the liver. Angiotensin I is subsequently converted to angiotensin II by angiotensin-converting enzyme (ACE), which is found in the lung, in the vascular endothelial cell luminal membrane, and locally in the glomerulus.[2] Over the past 40 years, it has been recognized that there are renal and other extrarenal RAS pathways leading to angiotensin II synthesis located in the brain, vascular endothelium, and adrenal gland. It is speculated that such systems are important in the regulation of vascular injury and repair responses.

Locally synthesized angiotensin II in the vascular endothelium and that generated by the kidneys may play a pivotal role in the development of hypertension by regulation of vascular tone, renal vasoconstriction, and sodium retention.

Division of Nephrology, Department of Medicine, University of Maryland School of Medicine, 22 S. Greene Street, N3W143, Baltimore, MD 21201, USA
* Corresponding author.
E-mail address: mweir@medicine.umaryland.edu (M.R. Weir).

Clin Geriatr Med 25 (2009) 245–257
doi:10.1016/j.cger.2009.01.007
0749-0690/09/$ – see front matter © 2009 Elsevier Inc. All rights reserved.

geriatric.theclinics.com

It has been recognized that plasma renin activity falls with increasing age.[3] There-fore, it might be anticipated that the blood pressure response to RAS inhibition may be reduced in older persons. In contrast, Ajayi and colleagues demonstrated greater blood pressure control with enalapril and intravenous enalaprilat in the older popula-tion (age, 65–73 years) compared with that in the younger population (22–30 years).[15]

Physiologic aging is associated with increased angiotensin II production in arterial tissue. This may explain the age-related decrease in endothelial function in the healthy older population.[4] The localized angiotensin II production may explain the beneficial effect of RAS inhibition even in older patients with low circulating angiotensin II levels or plasma renin activity.[2] In recent years, the pathophysiological implications of the RAS pathway has been a major focus of attention, and inhibitors of the RAS such as ACE inhibitors, angiotensin II receptor blockers (ARBs), and direct renin inhibitors have become important clinical tools in the treatment of blood pressure and cardio-vascular and renal diseases.[1]

RENIN ANGIOTENSIN SYSTEM AND AGING

Older persons in better health have a longer life expectancy than that of persons in poorer health, yet they have similar cumulative health care expenditures until death. A person with no functional limitation at 70 years of age has a life expectancy of 14.3 years and expected cumulative health care expenditures of about $136,000 (in 1998 dollars).[5] It makes important sense to focus on ways of diminishing the morbidity and mortality of cardiovascular disease, especially in the healthy, older population. Aging is strongly correlated with endothelial dysfunction in animals and humans.[6] Mukai and colleagues[7] have demonstrated that long-term inhibition of the RAS ameliorates the endothelial dysfunction associated with aging by inhibiting the synthesis of cyclooxygenase related vasoconstriction factors and superoxide anions. Will this effect prove helpful in reducing the risks of vascular disease? Will RAS inhibi-tion in the older population have a different effect compared with that in younger persons on the different vascular pathologic processes that are more prevalent with aging? What age is the cutoff for dichotomizing the population into older versus younger, given that age and life expectancy are moving targets? Although there are numerous studies addressing different questions and multiple prevalent diseases, such as diabetes mellitus and cardiovascular and kidney diseases, few target the older population (Fig. 1).This is partly due to the ethical dimension that is placed to protect this more fragile population with multiple comorbidities, which could possibly confound clinical trials. Hence, most of the data used in this review were extracted from trials that had an average age of 65 years, with a lower age limit of 55 years and an upper age limit of 80 years.

RAS INHIBITION ADVANTAGES IN OLDER PATIENTS
Congestive Heart Failure

A meta-analysis of 32 randomized, controlled trials by Garg and Yusuf in 7105 patients, with advanced New York Heart Association functional class II or worse and ejection fraction less than 0.35 to 0.4 with or without limitation of exercise, concluded that ACE inhibitors reduced total mortality (odds ratio, 0.77; 95% confidence interval [CI], 0.67–0.88; $P<.001$) and the combined risk of mortality and hospitalization for conges-tive heart failure (CHF). When these patients were dichotomized based on age less than or greater than 60 years, there was no observable difference in the benefits of ACE inhibitor on all-cause mortality. In the Effect of Enalapril on Survival in Patients with reduced Left Ventricular Ejection Fraction (Studies of Left Ventricular Dysfunction) trial

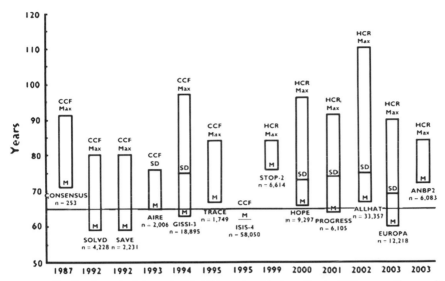

Fig. 1. Age distribution of trials on ACE inhibitors in elderly patients. CCF, congestive cardiac failure; HCR, high cardiovascular risk; M, mean age; Max, maximum age; SD, standard deviation. (*From* Mangoni AA, Jackson SH. The implications of a growing evidence base for drug use in elderly patients Part 2. ACE inhibitors and angiotensin receptor blockers in heart failure and high cardiovascular risk patients. Br J Clin Pharmacol 2006;61(5):502–12; with permission.)

(mean age, 60 years) addition of enalapril significantly reduced morbidity and mortality in patients with CHF.[8] The effect of enalapril on 12-year survival and life expectancy follow-up in patients with and without symptomatic left ventricular dysfunction demonstrated that, compared with placebo, enalapril equally improved long-term survival in persons younger and older than 61 years of age.[9]

The Survival and Ventricular Enlargement (SAVE) Trial, which investigated the effect of captopril versus placebo on morbidity and mortality in patients with left ventricular dysfunction post myocardial infarction patients, demonstrated that all-cause mortality was significantly reduced and a greater benefit observed in patients aged 65 years and older.[10]

In a retrospective study of an older population with CHF, where the mean age was 85 years, The Systematic Assessment of Geriatric Drug Use via Epidemiology study group demonstrated a 10% reduction in the mortality rate among the cohort that used ACE inhibitors in comparison with the group that used digoxin.[11] However, the question of efficacy of ACE inhibitors among older patients with asymptomatic left ventricular dysfunction remains controversial.[12]

The efficacy of ACE inhibitors and ARBs in reducing cardiovascular morbidity and mortality in older patients with heart failure has been established. The effect of ACE inhibition—angiotensin receptor blockade—or a combination regimen on events in older persons postmyocardial infarction complicated by left ventricular dysfunction has been investigated by Pfeffer and colleagues[10] in a double blind, placebo-controlled (Valsartan in Acute Myocardial Infarction trial) trial, with a mean age of 64.8 ± 11.8 years. This trial compared the effect of valsartan, captopril, or both on cardiovascular outcomes and demonstrated that valsartan is as effective as captopril in improving survival and reducing cardiovascular morbidity among patients with high cardiovascular risk after myocardial infarction. However, combination therapy did not show any advantage in reducing mortality or cardiovascular morbidity and mortality. The beneficial effect of both valsartan and captopril was similar in patients older as well as younger than 65 years of age.

Angiotensin II, which is a potent vasoconstrictor and growth-stimulating hormone contributes to progression of heart failure. The long-term effect of adding an ARB valsartan to patients with heart failure was evaluated by Cohn and colleagues[13] in a randomized, placebo-controlled, double-blind, parallel-group trial, of patients with a mean age of 62 years. Valsartan reduced combined morbidity and mortality incidence by 13.2% compared with placebo (relative risk, 0.87; 97.5% CI, 0.77–0.97; $P = .009$) and improved clinical signs and symptoms of heart failure. The beneficial effect of valsartan was consistent among older as well as younger persons.

Whether ARB alone, or with ACE inhibitor, is effective in managing older patients with heart failure has been investigated by Pfeffer and colleagues[14] by studying the effect of candesartan on mortality and morbidity in patients with chronic heart failure (Candesartan in Heart Failure-Assessment of Reduction in Mortality and Morbidity overall program). This study was a randomized, double-blind, placebo-controlled trial in patients with a mean age of 65 years. Candesartan was well tolerated, and it reduced cardiovascular morbidity and mortality irrespective of baseline ejection fraction or type of treatment. Similarly, patients aged 75 years and older demonstrated as much benefit with candesartan as did younger patients. Thus, these data demonstrate that RAS blockade in persons with and without symptomatic heart failure provides comparable mortality and morbidity benefits across all age groups, including patients older than 75 years.

Hypertension

Hypertension is a major risk factor for coronary artery disease, stroke, and progression of diabetes-related kidney disease in older persons. As the number of older individuals increases among the general population, it is important to note that the risk of medication-related adverse outcomes also increases with age. Thus, more studies are needed to evaluate the risks and benefits of different antihypertensive therapies such as RAS inhibitors in older persons. Unfortunately, most of the studies are performed in younger populations.[15] There is continued debate over which antihypertensive medication is most appropriate as a first-line therapy in the older population. In the past, thiazide diuretics have been recommended as the preferred agents (The Seventh Report of the Joint National Committee on Prevention, Detection, Evaluation, and Treatment of High Blood Pressure). However, since older persons often have multiple medical comorbidities, other agents such as RAS inhibitors are an important consideration. Hypertension in older persons is characterized by increased peripheral resistance and decreased arterial compliance. RAS blockade leads to dilatation of small and large arteries, which helps correct these 2 age-related pathophysiological changes.[16] Plasma renin activity is known to fall in older populations, yet some studies have demonstrated that ACE inhibitors lead to greater fall in blood pressure in older patients compared with that in younger patients. In a single-blind, placebo-controlled, randomized, crossover study in normotensive healthy young (22–30 years) and older (65–73 years) persons, both enalapril and intravenous enalaprilat were found to reduce blood pressure effectively. The decrease in blood pressure was numerically greater in the older group. However, this study was limited by the small number of subjects used, and baseline blood pressure was higher in the older population.[15] However, not all studies showed the same results. Some feel that RAS inhibitors may be more effective in younger rather than in older populations.[16]

In the Antihypertensive and Lipid Lowering Treatment to Prevent Heart Attack Trial (ALLHAT), which included patients who were 55 years of age or older, chlorthalidone and lisinopril were found to have similar efficacy for reducing the primary endpoint of all-cause, fatal, and nonfatal coronary heart disease (CHD) events (relative risk (RR), 0.99; 95% CI, 0.91–1.08) and the secondary outcomes of all-cause mortality, combined CHD, peripheral arterial disease, and end stage renal disease (ESRD). Nonetheless, the conclusion of the study was that thiazide-type diuretics (chlorthalidone) were superior in preventing one or more of the cardiovascular outcomes in comparison to the ACE inhibitor (lisinopril). This conclusion was likely based on the higher overall risk for stroke and combined cardiovascular events in the lisinopril group compared with that in the diuretic group, because patients on chlorthalidone had their blood pressure much more effectively controlled than did the patients on lisinopril.[17] However, older patients will likely require two or more drugs to lower their blood pressure, and thiazides are quite effective in lowering blood pressure with RAS-blocking drugs such as ACE and ARB.

The Losartan Intervention for Endpoint Reduction (LIFE) study, which was a double-blind, randomized trial, compared losartan and atenolol plus other medications in older patients with isolated systolic hypertension (ISH) (mean age, 70 years). The mean sitting systolic blood pressure was reduced by 28 mm Hg in both losartan and atenolol regimens. However, patients who were on losartan had 25% relative risk reduction (RRR) in cardiovascular death, stroke, and myocardial infarction. Thus, this trial showed that the RAS-blocking regimen is superior to a beta-blocking regimen in reducing cardiovascular events with ISH in older patients.[18]

Although RAS-blocking drugs are well tolerated, in older populations, they will often need to be combined with other drugs such as thiazide diuretics or calcium channel blockers to help reduce systolic blood pressure. Since systolic blood pressure is the most important treatment variable in older populations, more trials are needed to establish which drugs are best to use with RAS inhibitors to both lower pressure and cardiovascular events. The recently published Avoiding Cardiovascular Events in Combination Therapy in Patients Living with Systolic Hypertension (ACCOMPLISH)[19] study suggests that calcium channel blocker when combined with RAS-blocking therapy may have some advantages in older populations with cardiovascular risk factors.

Cardiovascular Disease

In The Heart Outcomes Prevention Evaluation Study, 9,297 high-risk subjects (age, 55 years or older) with high risk for cardiovascular events (without left ventricular dysfunction) were randomized to treatment with ramipril versus placebo in addition to their current cardiovascular-risk-reducing therapy. Ramipril treatment reduced the rates of death from cardiovascular disease (RR, 0.74; $P<.001$), myocardial infarction (RR, 0.8; $P<.001$), revascularization (RR, 0.85; $P=.002$), cardiac arrest (RR, 0.63; $P=.03$), and heart failure (RR, 0.77; $P<.001$) compared with placebo. However, there was also a 3/2 mm Hg blood pressure advantage in the ramipril treatment group.[20] Thus, RAS inhibition does help in older populations. Similar results were observed in the The Ongoing Telmisartan Alone and in Combination with Ramipril Global Endpoint Trial study when an ACE inhibitor-based or an ARB-based antihypertensive regimen was compared on cardiovascular events in an older population with risk factors for cardiovascular disease.[21]

Hypertension is a well-documented risk factor for myocardial infarction, heart failure, and atherosclerosis. In a secondary analysis of the SAVE trial, the investigators evaluated the efficacy of captopril versus placebo in younger and older patients (age, more than 60 years) who survived a myocardial infarction. The overall incidence of combined cardiovascular events, such as heart failure, fatal and nonfatal recurrent myocardial infarction, and cardiovascular and all-cause death, was less in the captopril group in comparison with that in the placebo group in both hypertensive and normotensive patients.[12] Greater benefit was observed in patients who were older than 65 years (absolute risk reduction 8.2%).

Not all studies have demonstrated the benefit of RAS inhibition in the secondary prevention of CHD. These conflicting results may be explained by the age difference in the different trial populations. Trials that enrolled older persons demonstrated the beneficial effect of ACE-inhibitor therapy in secondary prevention of CHD, because older patients had greater cardiovascular risk and higher mean blood pressure.[22] Thus, some of the most consistent data with RAS inhibition benefits on cardiovascular disease are observed in older populations.

Cerebrovascular Disease

Effective blood pressure control is beneficial in reducing the risk of stroke. However, there is limited evidence of benefit in treating patients 80 years of age and older. Most previous studies either excluded patients older than 80 years, or the number of subjects enrolled was small. In the Hypertension in the Very Elderly Trial, which included only hypertensive patients who were 80 years of age or older, patients were randomized to receive indapamide alone, or with perindopril, versus placebo. The goal blood pressure with treatment was 150/80 mm Hg. Those who were in the active treatment group demonstrated a 30% reduction in the rate of fatal and nonfatal cerebrovascular accidents (95% CI, -1 to 51; P = .06) and a 39% reduction in the rate of death from stroke. More importantly, there was no significant change in baseline serum potassium level or creatinine between the two groups. The investigators concluded that even older patients, older than 80 years, derive benefit with antihypertensive therapy using thiazide diuretics with or without ACE inhibitors.[23]

In the ALLHAT trial, the importance of blood pressure control on stroke prevention was evident. Patients who received lisinopril demonstrated a higher risk of stroke in comparison to the group on chlorthalidone (6.3% versus 5.6%; RR, 1.15; 95% CI, 1.02–1.30). This important difference was attributed to lower blood pressure attained in the chlorthalidone group compared with that in the lisinopril group (**Fig. 2**). In a randomized, double-blind, placebo-controlled trial (Perindopril Protection Against Recurrent Stroke Study [PROGRESS]) in patients with a prior history of cerebrovascular accident or transient ischemic attack, with a mean age 64 years, treatment with perindopril (4 mg/d) with or without the use of a diuretic (indapamide) was found to decrease the risk of stroke. The investigators concluded that combination therapy with RAS blockade and a diuretic reduces the risk of stroke recurrence among hypertensive patients.[24,25]

In the LIFE trial, the ARB-based regimen demonstrated a reduction in nonfatal and fatal stroke, cardiovascular mortality, all-cause mortality, and new-onset diabetes compared with a beta–blocker-based antihypertensive regimen. The majority of patients had systolic hypertension and left ventricular hypertrophy, which is a major risk factor for stroke. This study provided more evidence that RAS blockade (with an ARB) provides an important opportunity to reduce the risk of stroke in older persons. In summary, blood pressure control with the use of RAS blockade and other drugs in older populations reduces the risk of stroke and its related disabilities.

Left Ventricular Hypertrophy

The prevalence of Left ventricular hypertrophy (LVH) increases with age. It is known that angiotensin II plays a role in development of LVH. LVH prevalence by echocardiography is common and is found in 33% of men and 49% of women by the time they are 70 years or older.[26] LVH is recognized to be an independent predictor for CHD events,

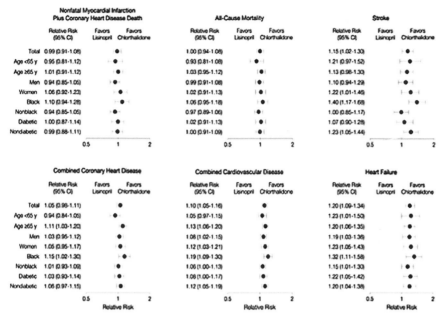

Fig. 2. Relative risks and 95% confidence intervals for lisinopril/chlorthalidone comparisons in prespecified subgroups. (*From* ALLHAT Officers and Coordinators for the ALLHAT Collaborative Research Group. Major outcomes in high-risk hypertensive patients randomized to angiotensin-converting enzyme inhibitor or calcium channel blocker vs diuretic: The Antihypertensive and Lipid-Lowering Treatment to Prevent Heart Attack Trial (ALLHAT). JAMA 2002;288(23):2981–97; with permission.)

heart failure, and cerebrovascular accidents. In a meta-analysis of double-blind, randomized, controlled trials, LVH regression occurred in 13% of patients receiving ARB, 11% with calcium channel blockers, 10% with ACE inhibitors, 8% with diuretics, and 6% with beta-receptor blockers.[27]

Secondary analyses of clinical trials demonstrate that regression of LVH is associated with reduced cardiovascular risk. The LIFE study (previously discussed) evaluated the long-term effect of the ARB losartan in comparison to the beta-blocker atenolol in older patients with LVH. The investigators noted that losartan was more effective than atenolol in reducing LVH. Despite similar changes in blood pressure, the losartan-based regimen was associated with 25% RRR in the cardiovascular mortality, fatal and nonfatal stroke, and total mortality.[18] Thus, RAS blockade with similar blood pressure reduction in older persons results in LVH regression and a reduction as that seen with beta blockade of cardiovascular and stroke mortality.[28]

Chronic Kidney Disease and Diabetic Nephropathy

With aging, chronic diseases, including chronic kidney disease (CKD), are expected to increase with a resultant rise in disability and financial burden on the health care system.[29] For example, in the National Health and Nutrition Examination Survey database, the prevalence of CKD increases with age, such that the prevalence for stage 3 to 4 CKD increases from 27.8% to 37.8% after the age of 70 years.[30]

The ALLHAT study did not demonstrate differences in the rate of CKD progression based on whether the patients were treated with diuretic, calcium channel blocker, or ACE inhibitor. However, the study did not enroll patients with kidney disease and lacked the power to evaluate the possible differences between therapies. The Ramipril Efficacy in Nephropathy study was a prospective evaluation of 322 patients with nondiabetic renal disease and proteinuria who were treated with the ACE inhibitor, ramipril, or placebo. Ramipril treatment slowed the progression of renal disease. The renoprotective and dialysis-saving effects were independent of the severity of kidney disease.[29] However, most of the patients were younger than 65 years of age with a median age of 50 years. During the study period, those with proteinuria less than 2 g/24 h of protein or polycystic kidney disease did not benefit by treatment to an appreciable extent.[31]

The Reduction of Endpoints in NIDDM with Angiotensin II Antagonist Losartan (RENAAL) study compared a losartan-based regimen and a placebo-based regimen in patients with type 2 diabetes with nephropathy. The average patient age was 60 years. The patients were followed for a mean period of 3.5 years. The study demonstrated that the ARB-based regimen (losartan) reduced the risk of serum creatinine doubling by 25% and (ESRD) by 28% independent of blood pressure reduction.[32] This benefit was observed regardless of age. The Irbesartan Diabetic Nephropathy trial had a similar age distribution as that of the RENAAL study, with an average age just under 60 years. In this study, three different blood pressure lowering regimens, amlodipine-based, irbesartan-based, or placebo-based multiple drug regimens, were used in a randomized design in patients with type 2 diabetes and nephropathy. As in the RENAAL study, the irbesartan-based therapy slowed diabetic nephropathy progression by increasing the time to serum creatinine doubling, ESRD, and all-cause cardiovascular events compared with the other regimens.[33] The results of these studies clearly demonstrate the utility of RAS blockade (either ACE inhibitor or ARB, depending on the study) to prevent progression of renal disease even in older populations. We suspect that this benefit is evident regardless of age, even though none of these studies purposely studied patients older than 75 years.

In a multinational, randomized, double-blind, placebo-controlled trial, the added benefit of RAS inhibition by using a direct renin inhibitor (aliskiren) and an ARB (losartan) was evaluated in both young and older individuals with type 2 diabetes complicated by nephropathy and hypertension (subjects ages ranged from 18–85 years with a mean of ∼60 years). The trial demonstrated that RAS inhibition using both a renin inhibitor and ARB had a greater antiproteinuric effect than the ARB alone, independent of the blood pressure lowering effect.[34] Thus, this type of dual RAS inhibition may be useful in older populations.

Physical Performance

It has been recognized that there is an age-related decline in physical function and exercise capacity. This decline eventually leads to disability in the older population. The functional decline is usually caused by underlying comorbidities, that is, stroke, CHF, and chronic degenerative joint disease, or sometimes may be related to cognitive functional decline. Onder and colleagues theorized that ACE inhibitors have direct metabolic and mechanical effects on skeletal muscle by affecting the myosin heavy chain. This stimulates the conversion of muscle fibers to a slow, aerobic, and fatigue-resistant isoform. Moreover, ACE inhibition augments muscle sensitivity to insulin and glycogen storage. An increase in kinins, as a result of ACE inhibition, is thought to enhance skeletal-muscle blood flow through its vasodilator effect.[35]

It is also speculated that an inhibitory effect of ACE inhibitors on the inflammatory mediators, interleukin-6, and tumor necrosis factor-α, could improve muscle function and decrease disability.[36] Graziano and colleagues evaluated the effects of ACE inhibition in an observational study on muscle strength in 755 hypertensive women with an average age 78.9 years. They were selected from the Women's Health and Aging Study population. They observed that treatment with an ACE inhibitor may decrease or stop the deterioration of muscle strength in older women with hypertension.[35]

Another smaller trial (n = 95), mean age 78.8 years, studied older patients with the ACE inhibitor perindopril or placebo. The trial demonstrated that perindopril significantly improved exercise capacity in functionally limited older subjects who had no CHF. As a result of this improvement, they were able to maintain health-related quality of life (**Fig. 3**).[37] ACE inhibition is also known to reduce physical function decline in older persons with CHF.[11,35]

In summary, there is evidence of positive association between RAS blockade and muscle-function improvement in the older patients. This improvement may hinder health-related quality-of-life deterioration. ACE inhibitors have multiple functional beneficial effects on muscle function. Whether ARB has a comparable beneficial effect needs further evaluation.[38] Future clinical trials with longer follow-up are needed to establish the durability of improvement and impact on survival.

Cognitive Impairment

With increasing life expectancy, the prevalence of vascular and Alzheimer's dementia is expected to increase from 33 million in 2007 to 81.1 million by 2040. There is substantial evidence that antihypertensive drug therapy reduces the incidence of dementia and cognitive impairment.[8] On the other hand, hypertension and stroke are associated with increased risk of vascular dementia in older persons.[39] There is an interest in evaluating the effect of RAS blockade on the risk of dementia, as an ACE-gene insertion deletion polymorphism is implicated in Alzheimer's dementia pathogenesis.[40] ACE is overexpressed in the hippocampus, frontal cortex, and caudate nucleus of patients with Alzheimer's disease.[41] Thus, targeting the RAS may be of benefit in older persons at risk of dementia.

In a randomized, prospective trial 162 older, long-term facility residents with hypertension (BP >140/90 mm Hg), with mild-moderate Alzheimer's dementia, and aged 65 years and older, patients were randomized to a brain-penetrating ACE inhibitor, a non–brain-penetrating ACE inhibitor, or a calcium channel blocker. The investigators

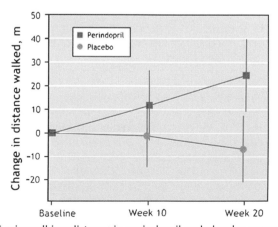

Fig. 3. Change in 6-min walking distance in perindopril and placebo groups from baseline to 10 wk and 20 wk. (*From* Sumukadas D, Witham MD, Struthers AD, McMurdo ME. Effect of perindopril on physical function in elderly people with functional impairment: a randomized controlled trial. CMAJ 2007;177(8):867–74; with permission.)

demonstrated slower mean 1-year decline in the Mini Mental State Examination score in the brain-penetrating ACE inhibitor-regimen group (0.6 ± 0.1) in comparison with the non–brain-penetrating ACE inhibitor-regimen (4.6 ± 0.3) and calcium channel blocker-regimen (4.9 ± 0.3) groups.[41] The Perindopril Protection Against Recurrent Stroke Study (PROGRESS) was a double-blind, placebo-controlled trial (n = 6105), with patients with a mean age of 64 years. Patients with previous stroke or transient ischemic attack were randomized to a perindopril, perindopril and indapamide, or matching placebo regimen. The study demonstrated that patients receiving the ACE inhibitor, perindopril, had a lower risk of dementia and progression of their cognitive decline associated with recurrent stroke.[39] In the SCOPE trial, patients aged 70 to 89 years with systolic hypertension (160–179 mm Hg) were randomized to receive candesartan or placebo. During the study, the investigators noted that there was more blood pressure reduction with candesartan-based therapy, but there was no difference in cognitive decline or dementia development observed between the candesartan or placebo groups. Unfortunately, only 25% of the active treatment group were taking their originally assigned regimen, which likely limits the interpretability of the results.[42] Thus, apart from high blood pressure control, RAS blockade may play a direct role in reducing the risk of Alzheimer's dementia and cognitive decline in older patients. Whether one category of antihypertensive drug, and particularly the RAS blockers, is more effective in slowing cognitive decline and development of dementia compared with other drugs is unknown.[43]

RAS INHIBITION LIMITATIONS IN OLDER PATIENTS

In the medical community, there is concern that RAS inhibition in older persons may aggravate the risk of hypotension, which could lead to increased risk of fall. Other concerns about RAS inhibition include reduction in kidney function, hyperkalemia, angioedema, and cough. The results of multiple studies do not support these concerns, as the risk of adverse events does not appear to be different in older persons compared with that in younger persons. In fact, the overall incidence of serious adverse events is often lower in patients on RAS inhibitors (4.6%/6.6%).[18] Studies with RAS inhibitors in older hypertensive patients do not show an increased risk of side effects despite effective blood pressure reduction.[15] Even combining diuretics with RAS inhibitors in older patients does not appear to increase the risk of changes in serum creatinine or potassium.[23] In general, the data for clinical trials demonstrate no evidence that age plays a role in the risk of adverse events with RAS inhibitor drugs.

SUMMARY

RAS inhibitors are effective and well-tolerated antihypertensive drugs for older persons. The efficacy and safety of these drugs are also evident in older persons even in the presence of CHF, LVH, and left ventricular dysfunction.[12] There is evidence that the RAS plays an important role in the pathobiology of vascular disease among the older population.[22] These drugs should be considered routinely in older populations due to their tolerability and cardiovascular benefits. Individualized use of these drugs is necessary to properly adjust the dose and use them in conjunction with other drugs.

ACKNOWLEDGMENTS

We thank Tia A. Paul, University of Maryland School of Medicine, Baltimore, MD, for editing the manuscript.

REFERENCES

1. Paul M, Poyan Mehr A, Kreutz R. Physiology of local renin-angiotensin systems. Physiol Rev 2006;86:747–803.
2. Rose BD, Post T. Renal circulation and glomerular filtration rate. Clinical physiology of acid base & electrolyte disorder. New York: McGraw-Hill; 2001.
3. Meade TW, Imeson JD, Gordon D, et al. The epidemiology of plasma renin. Clin Sci (Lond) 1983;64:273–80.
4. Macías Núñez JF. The aging kidney in health and disease. New York: Springer Science; 2008. p. 273.
5. Lubitz J, Cai L, Kramarow E, et al. Health, life expectancy, and health care spending among the elderly. N Engl J Med 2003;349:1048–55.
6. Matz RL, Schott C, Stoclet JC, et al. Age-related endothelial dysfunction with respect to nitric oxide, endothelium-derived hyperpolarizing factor and cyclooxygenase products. Physiol Res 2000;49:11–8.
7. Mukai Y, Shimokawa H, Higashi M, et al. Inhibition of renin-angiotensin system ameliorates endothelial dysfunction associated with aging in rats. Arterioscler Thromb Vasc Biol 2002;22:1445–50.
8. Poon I. Effect of enalapril on survival in patients with reduced left ventricular ejection fractions and congestive heart failure. The SOLVD Investigators. N Engl J Med 1991;325:293–302.
9. Jong P, Yusuf S, Rousseau MF, et al. Effect of enalapril on 12-year survival and life expectancy in patients with left ventricular systolic dysfunction: a follow-up study. Lancet 2003;361:1843–8.
10. Pfeffer MA, McMurray JJ, Velazquez EJ, et al. Valsartan, captopril, or both in myocardial infarction complicated by heart failure, left ventricular dysfunction, or both. N Engl J Med 2003;349:1893–906.
11. Gambassi G, Lapane KL, Sgadari A, et al. Effects of angiotensin-converting enzyme inhibitors and digoxin on health outcomes of very old patients with heart failure. SAGE Study Group. Systematic assessment of geriatric drug use via epidemiology. Arch Intern Med 2000;160:53–60.
12. Mangoni AA, Jackson SH. The implications of a growing evidence base for drug use in elderly patients Part 2. ACE inhibitors and angiotensin receptor blockers in heart failure and high cardiovascular risk patients. Br J Clin Pharmacol 2006;61:502–12.
13. Cohn JN, Tognoni G, the Valsartan Heart Failure Trial Investigators. A randomized trial of the angiotensin-receptor blocker valsartan in chronic heart failure. N Engl J Med 2001;345:1667–75.
14. Pfeffer MA, Swedberg K, Granger CB, et al. Effects of candesartan on mortality and morbidity in patients with chronic heart failure: the CHARM-Overall programme. Lancet 2003;362:759–66.
15. Ajayi AA, Hockings N, Reid JL. Age and the pharmacodynamics of angiotensin converting enzyme inhibitors enalapril and enalaprilat. Br J Clin Pharmacol 1986;21:349–57.
16. Forette F, McClaran J, Delesalle MC, et al. Value of angiotensin converting enzyme inhibitors in the elderly: the example of perindopril. Clin Exp Hypertens A 1989;11(Suppl 2):587–603.
17. The ALLHAT Officers and Coordinators for the ALLHAT Collaborative Research Group. Major outcomes in high-risk hypertensive patients randomized to angiotensin-converting enzyme inhibitor or calcium channel blocker vs diuretic: The Antihypertensive and Lipid-Lowering Treatment to Prevent Heart Attack Trial (ALLHAT). JAMA 2002;288:2981–97.

18. Kjeldsen SE, Dahlof B, Devereux RB, et al. Effects of losartan on cardiovascular morbidity and mortality in patients with isolated systolic hypertension and left ventricular hypertrophy: A Losartan Intervention For Endpoint Reduction (LIFE) Substudy. JAMA 2002;288:1491–8.
19. Jamerson K, Weber MA, Bakris GL, et al. Benazepril plus amlodipine or hydrochlorothiazide for hypertension in high-risk patients. N Engl J Med 2008;359:2417–28.
20. Yusuf S, Sleight P, Pogue J, et al. Effects of an angiotensin-converting-enzyme inhibitor, ramipril, on cardiovascular events in high-risk patients. The Heart Outcomes Prevention Evaluation Study Investigators. N Engl J Med 2000;342:145–53.
21. ONTARGET Investigators, Yusuf S, Teo KK, et al. Telmisartan, ramipril, or both in patients at high risk for vascular events. N Engl J Med 2008;358(15):1547–59.
22. Hammoud RA, Vaccari CS, Nagamia SH, et al. Regulation of the renin-angiotensin system in coronary atherosclerosis: a review of the literature. Vasc Health Risk Manag 2007;3:937–45.
23. Beckett NS, Peters R, Fletcher AE, et al. Treatment of hypertension in patients 80 years of age or older. N Engl J Med 2008;358:1887–98.
24. PROGRESS. Randomised trial of a perindopril-based blood-pressure lowering regimen among individuals with previous stroke or transient ischaemic attack. Lancet 2001;358:1033–41.
25. PROGRESS. Effects of a perindopril-based blood pressure-lowering regimen on disability and dependency in 6105 patients with cerebrovascular disease: A Randomized Controlled Trial. Stroke 2003;34:2333–8.
26. Levy D, Anderson KM, Savage DD, et al. Echocardiographically detected left ventricular hypertrophy: prevalence and risk factors. The Framingham Heart Study. Ann Intern Med 1988;108:7–13.
27. Klingbeil AU, Schneider M, Martus P, et al. A meta-analysis of the effects of treatment on left ventricular mass in essential hypertension. Am J Med 2003;115:41–6.
28. Dahlof B, Devereux R, de FU, et al. The losartan intervention for endpoint reduction (LIFE) in hypertension study: rationale, design, and methods. The LIFE Study Group. Am J Hypertens 1997;10:705–13.
29. Ruggenenti P, Perna A, Remuzzi G. ACE Inhibitors to prevent end-stage renal disease: when to start and why possibly never to stop: A Post Hoc Analysis of the REIN Trial Results. J Am Soc Nephrol 2001;12:2832–7.
30. Coresh J, Selvin E, Stevens LA, et al. Prevalence of chronic kidney disease in the United States. JAMA 2007;298:2038–47.
31. Ruggenenti P, Perna A, Zoccali C, et al. Chronic proteinuric nephropathies. II. Outcomes and response to treatment in a prospective cohort of 352 patients: differences between women and men in relation to the ACE gene polymorphism. J Am Soc Nephrol 2000;11:88–96.
32. Brenner BM, Cooper ME, de Zeeuw D, et al. Effects of losartan on renal and cardiovascular outcomes in patients with type 2 diabetes and nephropathy. N Engl J Med 2001;345:861–9.
33. Lewis EJ, Hunsicker LG, Clarke WR, et al. Renoprotective effect of the angiotensin-receptor antagonist irbesartan in patients with nephropathy due to type 2 diabetes. N Engl J Med 2001;345:851–60.
34. Parving HH, Persson F, Lewis JB, et al, the ASI. Aliskiren combined with losartan in type 2 diabetes and nephropathy. N Engl J Med 2008;358:2433–46.
35. Onder G, Penninx BW, Balkrishnan R, et al. Relation between use of angiotensin-converting enzyme inhibitors and muscle strength and physical function in older women: an observational study. Lancet 2002;359:926–30.

36. Cohen HJ, Pieper CF, Harris T, et al. The association of plasma IL-6 levels with functional disability in community-dwelling elderly. J Gerontol A Biol Sci Med Sci 1997;52:M201–8.
37. Sumukadas D, Witham MD, Struthers AD, et al. Effect of perindopril on physical function in elderly people with functional impairment: a randomized controlled trial. CMAJ 2007;177:867–74.
38. Carter CS, Onder G, Kritchevsky SB, et al. Angiotensin-converting enzyme inhibition intervention in elderly persons: effects on body composition and physical performance. J Gerontol A Biol Sci Med Sci 2005;60:1437–46.
39. Tzourio C, Anderson C, Chapman N, et al. Effects of blood pressure lowering with perindopril and indapamide therapy on dementia and cognitive decline in patients with cerebrovascular disease. Arch Intern Med 2003;163:1069–75.
40. Gustafson DR, Melchior L, Eriksson E, et al. The ACE insertion deletion polymorphism relates to dementia by metabolic phenotype, APOE[var epsilon]4, and age of dementia onset. Neurobiology of Aging 2008, in press.
41. Ohrui T, Tomita N, Sato-Nakagawa T, et al. Effects of brain-penetrating ACE inhibitors on Alzheimer disease progression. Neurology 2004;63:1324-5.
42. Lithell H, Hansson L, Skoog I, et al. The Study on Cognition and Prognosis in the Elderly (SCOPE): principal results of a randomized double-blind intervention trial. J Hypertens 2003;21:875–86.
43. Hanes DS, Weir MR. Usefulness of ARBs and ACE inhibitors in the prevention of vascular dementia in the elderly. Am J Geriatr Cardiol 2007;16:175–82.

Hypertension and Cognitive Function

Thomas Olabode Obisesan, MD, MPH*

KEYWORDS

- Aging • Memory • Dementia • Alzheimer's disease
- Hypertension • Prevention • Treatment

Advanced age is a key risk factor for dementia and hypertension (**Fig. 1**). By the year 2030, the number of individuals aged 60 years and older will reach 70 million in the United States alone.[1–3] Fortunately, in addition to increased life expectancy, Americans are retaining vigor well into their 80s and beyond. But with longevity comes increased weakening of neurocognitive function. In this review, the author discusses the evidence indicating that primary and secondary prevention of hypertension may be an important public health goal in the United States for preventing or delaying cognitive loss.

Stroke and Alzheimer-type dementia increase at comparable rates with advancing age. Vascular disease is emerging as an important risk factor for dementia and Alzheimer disease (AD). In addition to age, diabetes, hypercholesterolemia, and presence of an apolipoprotein E4 (ApoE4) allele, all characterized by vascular pathology, hypertension is now considered an important risk factor for the sporadic, prevalent form of AD.[4] Evidence from epidemiologic and prospective studies lends credence to this new paradigm: The Rotterdam population-based prospective study that examined approximately 8000 subjects aged 55 years and older for the frequency of lifetime risk for dementia and its subtypes, including AD, showed an increase in the prevalence of atherosclerosis in vascular dementia and AD.[5] Compilation of autopsy reports on AD brains indicates that approximately 60% to 90% of the cases exhibited variable cerebrovascular pathology synonymous with cerebrovascular disease (CVD).[6,7] In AD cases ascertained by the presence of amyloid angiopathy, endothelial degeneration, and periventricular white matter lesions at autopsy, Van Nostrand and colleagues[8] showed that approximately one-third had evidence of cerebral infarction. These reports indicate that CVD risk factors may also influence AD development.

From the CVD risk factors examined in many epidemiologic and clinical trials thus far, hypertension is recognized as the most consistent risk factor for stroke and, importantly, AD.[9–13] Hypertension-related silent ischemic white matter increases

Supported by grant numbers: AG00980 (TOO) from the National Institute of Health, and RO1 AG02213 (RCG) also from the National Institute of Health.
Division of Geriatrics, Department of Medicine, Howard University Hospital, 2041 Georgia Avenue, NW, Washington, DC 20060, USA
* Corresponding author.
E-mail address: tobisesan@howard.edu

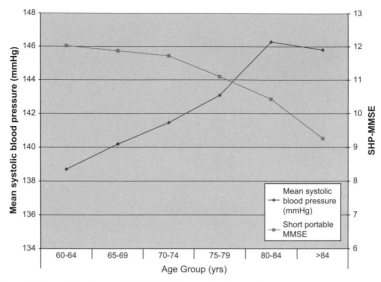

Fig. 1. Mean SBP and short portable MMSE score by increasing age groups.

with elevated blood pressure and is increasingly seen to coexist with AD. In addition to its role in vascular dementia, hypertension is now considered to have a causal relationship with dementia of the AD type.[14,15] This belief is emphasized by prospective studies linking high blood pressure in midlife to dementia in late life.[14,15]

In addition to a causal relationship of hypertension with future cognitive decline, hypertension also contributes to known AD endophenotypes, such as brain volume. Specifically, systolic blood pressure (SBP) and pulse pressure (PPR) are associated with medial temporal lobe atrophy, which is a hallmark of AD (especially when they coexist with white matter changes) in individual with late-onset dementia.[16] Although it was previously believed that hypertension-related cognitive decline was mediated directly through multiple brain infarcts, the new evidence indicates that hypertension can also act directly or synergistically with vascular disease to promote AD development.

Evidence about whether medication can attenuate hypertension-related cognitive decline is slowly emerging. Such studies range from epidemiologic (cross-sectional and prospective) studies to meta-analyses and clinical trials. Mechanisms by which hypertension influences cognitive function are also being investigated. Of significant interest is cerebral hypertension-induced vascular stiffness and consequent reduction in brain perfusion. Fortunately, treatment to reduce blood pressure can prevent arterial stiffness and improve cerebral perfusion, and thereby preserve cognitive dexterity. Conversely, excessive blood pressure reduction, especially in the aged, can cause cerebral hypoperfusion and cognitive loss. Therefore, identification of optimal blood pressure for best cognitive performance and reduction in AD risk is of considerable scientific, clinical, and public health interest.

Although consensus is lacking on what blood pressure levels offer the best beneficial effects on cognition, enough evidence exists to preliminarily guide treatment goals in older hypertensive patients.[17–22] Using the Seventh Joint National Committee on Prevention, Detection, Evaluation, and Treatment of High Blood Pressure criteria, target blood pressure that is beneficial to cognition should be in the normal range (<120/80 mm Hg) for (1) persons 75 years or younger, (2) persons 75 years or older with new-onset hypertension, and (3) persons with diabetes, irrespective of age. For persons 75 years or older who have chronic hypertension, blood pressure in the pre-hypertensive range (120–139 mm Hg) is likely to be beneficial to cognition. Regardless of duration and history of hypertension, target blood pressure that is beneficial to cognition in persons 80 years or older should also remain in the prehypertensive range.

Medications used to achieve blood pressure control have significant cognitively beneficial effects that are independent of blood pressure levels. Dihydropyridine calcium channel blockers (DHP-CCBs), angiotensin converting enzyme (ACE) inhibitors, angiotensin receptor blockers (ARBs), and potassium-sparing diuretics exert cognitively beneficial effects. Although the evidence is hardly definitive, conversely, non-DHP-CCBs seem to have an opposing effect, possibly contributing to cognitive deterioration. These recommendations need to be substantiated in the future through double-blind placebo-controlled clinical trials.

Given the high prevalence of hypertension in the United States, substantial cognitive gains might be realized from the optimization of blood pressure. Even if hypertension only results in a moderately increased AD rate or overall dementia, better treatment and optimization of blood pressure can have a significant public health impact in primary prevention of AD and vascular dementia.[10]

In this review, the current understanding of the relationship of hypertension to cognitive health is discussed. The review focuses on evidence gathered from various study types, from cross-sectional studies to prospective and randomized controlled clinical trials, and posited mechanisms that mediate this relationship.

EVIDENCE LINKING HYPERTENSION TO COGNITIVE FUNCTION
Cross-sectional Studies

Evidence
Hypertension is associated with diminished performance on tests of cognitive function. Initial support for this view came from epidemiologic studies. A few of these studies examined the relationship of blood pressure to cognitive loss in late life,[23–26] and most reported beneficial effects. Although many such studies used varying degrees of blood pressure to define hypertension, a cross-sectional but rigorous epidemiologic study used a representative sample of the noninstitutionalized United States population to test the hypothesis that elevated blood pressure is associated with lower cognitive function.[17] In accordance with the sixth report of the Joint National Committee on Prevention, Detection, Evaluation, and Treatment of High Blood Pressure (JNC VI)[27] used by Obisesan and colleagues,[17] categories of blood pressure were defined as given in the next paragraph and in **Table 1**.

For the regression analysis used in the study, blood pressure was considered normal if SBP was from is ≤129 mm Hg or diastolic blood pressure (DBP) is ≤85 mm Hg. These categorizations have since been revised in the seventh report of the Joint National Committee on Prevention, Detection, Evaluation, and Treatment of High Blood Pressure and even more so in the pending revised version. Results from this study indicate that in age groups 60 to 64, 65 to 69, and 70 to 74, optimal blood pressure (<120/80 mm Hg) was associated with best cognitive performance; severe hypertension was associated with the poorest performance in all age groups except the very old (≥80 years), in whom the pattern was reversed, showing the poorest performance in the optimal blood pressure group and the best in the moderate hypertension group (**Fig. 2**). In analyses additionally adjusted for important covariates, increasing JNC-VI stage of hypertension associated with worsening cognitive performance compared with normal blood pressure at ages older than 70 years. This

Table 1		
Ranges for the various blood pressure categories		
	Blood Pressure (mm Hg)	
Blood Pressure Categories	Systolic	Diastolic
Optimal	<120	<80
Normal	120–129	80–85
Prehypertension	130–139	86–89
Stage I hypertension	140–159	90–99
Stage II hypertension	160–179	100–109
Stage III hypertension	≥180	≥110

relationship appears less certain in the younger age group. From such studies having sufficient power to conduct age-stratified analysis, it is evident that the relationship of hypertension to cognitive function is susceptible to age effect.

In addition to reports from the third National Health and Nutrition Examination Survey (NHANES III) data, other epidemiologic studies have reported on the association of blood pressure with cognitive loss.[11–13,28–32] A retrospective study of 89 patients with presenile dementia followed up by necropsy showed that approximately one-half of the 46 patients with AD and 3 of 16 mixed dementia subjects had systolic pressure greater than 140 mm Hg.[28] Independent of resting clinical blood pressure, SBP and DBP reactivity also correlated with diminished performance on tests of immediate and delayed verbal memory and executive function.[26] Together, this initial evidence supports the view that hypertension can attenuate cognitive reserve. These findings add significantly to growing evidence that uncontrolled hypertension contributes to dementia risk as the population ages.

Can hypertension treatment attenuate dementia risk?

The degree to which blood pressure is controlled in hypertensive patients is a critical determinant of related cognitive outcomes.[25] Hypertensive patients whose blood pressure is poorly controlled have reduced performance on cognitive tests. Although the overall goal of the treatment of hypertension is to normalize blood pressure and reduce hypertension-related cognitive loss, cross-sectional data indicate that treatment of hypertension even without control can reduce its negative influence on cognition. Preliminary evidence supporting this view came from the NHANES III data showing that compared with persons with hypertension or with hypertension that is untreated and uncontrolled, treated but uncontrolled hypertension is associated with better cognitive performance even after discounting the effects of important co-variates.[17] In another study to examine the relationship of hypertension and blood pressure levels to cognition, individuals with high blood pressure failed to perform optimally on tests of nonverbal memory, motor speed, and manual dexterity, irrespective of prior diagnostic status.[25] In this study, persons with hypertension who had poorly controlled blood pressure were most vulnerable to difficulties in tests on perceptuo-motor speed and manual dexterity compared with the control.[25] Together, the cross-sectional evidence indicates that elevated blood pressure and hypertension cause cognitive loss when compared with optimal blood pressure or blood pressure in the normal range. Also, the maintenance of blood pressure in the normal range can attenuate hypertension-related cognitive loss (**Fig. 3**). These associations are independent of other common risk factors such as age, gender, ethnicity, education, income level, and history of stroke (**Fig. 4**).

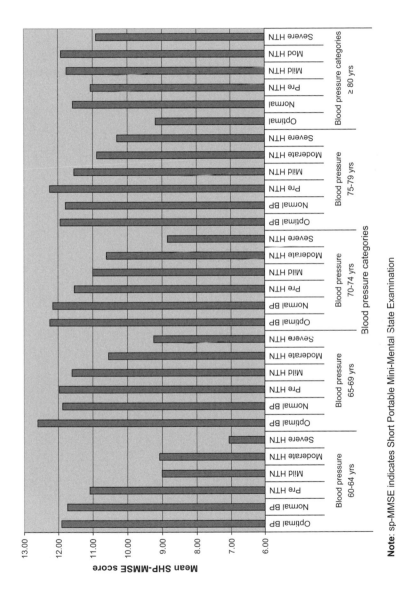

Note: sp-MMSE indicates Short Portable Mini-Mental State Examination

Fig. 2. Short portable MMSE score by JNC VI blood pressure categories in different age groups.

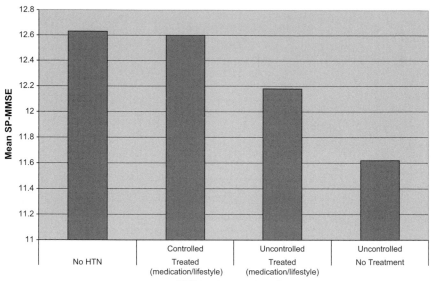

Note: Mean Short Portable Mini-Mental State Examination (sp-MMSE) score adjusted for age, gender, ethnicity, education, income, and pulse pressure.

Fig. 3. Short portable MMSE score by treatment categories.

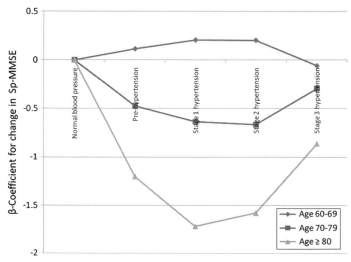

Note: optimal and normal are collapsed as one group; Sp-MMSE means short portable mini-mental state examination

Fig. 4. Age, gender, ethnicity, education, income, self-reported history of stroke and medication treatment, body mass index, glycosylated hemoglobin, and physical activity–adjusted change in short portable MMSE score according to JNC VI stages of blood pressure: The Third National Health and Nutrition Examination Survey (NHANES III).

Given these earlier observations, later epidemiologic work on the connection between blood pressure and cognitive function increasingly focuses on whether treatment with medication is beneficial in reducing hypertension-related cognitive loss. One such earlier report came from Cacciatore and colleagues,[33] who observed that hypertension treated with medication related to better cognitive outcome in an Italian sample. Building on the observation of Cacciatore and colleagues, Richards and colleagues[34] showed that hypertension treated with medication attenuated the related cognitive decline in a community sample of African Americans. As the evidence grew, interest also developed on whether the beneficial effect of treatment was because of a specific medication. In a study design similar to that of Richards and colleagues[34] that used a geriatric practice community sample, Hajjar and colleagues[35] provided additional insight by showing that the use of diuretics, β-blockers, and ACE inhibitors to treat hypertension associates with improved cognitive outcomes.

Jointly, this preliminary evidence indicates that cognitive outcomes in persons with hypertension whose blood pressure is controlled with medication and/or lifestyle alteration are similar to those in persons without hypertension; are slightly better than those in persons who underwent similar interventions but did not achieve blood pressure control; and are better than those in persons with hypertension not receiving treatment and whose blood pressure remained uncontrolled (see **Fig. 3**).[17] These findings support the need for increased attention to preventative efforts and maintenance of blood pressure in the normal range to preserve cognitive function.

Negative studies

Although most cross-sectional treatment studies on the relationship of hypertension to cognitive loss found that treatment is mostly beneficial, studies reporting negative findings merit a brief discussion. For example, the East Boston cohort study found no relationship of hypertension to cognitive function in nondemented persons.[36] In concordance with the East Boston study, a Canadian study on health and aging found no association of high blood pressure with cognitive decline or dementia.[37] Given that years of hypertension is required for the development of related cognitive loss later in life, a nonsignificant association of elevated blood pressure with performance on cognitive measures in studies involving a younger age group is logical. Alternatively, a lower prevalence of neurocognitive loss and AD in those aged less than 65 may also explain the negative findings. For studies involving an older age group, inadequate characterization of the sample and other bias inherent in cross-sectional studies are competing explanations.

Prospective Nonmedication Treatment Studies

In general, longitudinal studies are advantageous in that they provide information on the temporal relationship and the duration and the effect of chronic hypertension on cognitive function, especially given that years of sustained elevated blood pressure may be required for its effects on cognitive function (**Fig. 5**). A few such studies examined the effect of blood pressure on subsequent developments of cognitive loss, and most found an association of hypertension in midlife with neurocognitive loss about 15 to 20 years later.[38] For example, a significant association of hypertension with increased cognitive loss at follow-up was demonstrated in a sample of 700 patients with AD, who were followed for an average of 6 months.[39] These nonmedication prospective studies support observations from the initial cross-sectional studies that demonstrated the harmful effect of hypertension on cognition.

To further delineate the role of vascular disease, in particular hypertension, in the athogenesis of late-onset AD, Skoog and colleagues[13] analyzed the Longitudinal

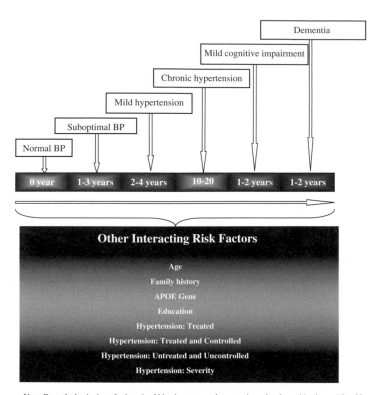

Note: From the beginning of sub-optimal blood pressure to hypertension-related cognitive loss, ~15 to 30 years may be required for its cognitive effects. Such effects will depend on the presence of other modifiers and or mediators such as: age, family history of AD, presence of APOE allele, gender, ethnicity, educational attainment, severity of hypertension, and whether or not hypertension is treated and or controlled.

Fig. 5. Time and sequence and interacting factors: Relationship of hypertension to future cognitive decline.

Population Study of 70-year-olds in Göteborg (Gothenburg), Sweden. In this study, persons with elevated blood pressure at about age 70 were more likely to have cognitive loss at ages 79 and 85 compared with controls. However, blood pressure differences between demented and nondemented groups tended to equilibrate in the years preceding the onset of actual cognitive loss,[13] a finding that is independently supported by the work of Hanon and colleagues[40] and Verghese and colleagues.[41] This finding led to the consideration that hypotension may be a clinical prodrome of AD.

After the initial characterization of mild cognitive impairment (MCI) as the prodromal stage of AD, its association with hypertension has also been a subject of debate. In a 21-year follow-up prospective Finnish population study to evaluate the impact of midlife elevated blood pressure on the subsequent development of MCI in the elderly, a tendency toward a significant relation between hypertension and the risk of MCI was observed.[11] Such observations in MCI patients support findings in demented patients.

If indeed hypertension is a risk factor for AD, it is reasonable to expect that it is also associated with important AD endophenotypes. To test this hypothesis, a population-based longitudinal study with 36 years of follow-up examined the relationship of midlife hypertension with later development of cognitive impairment, vascular dementia, and AD in Japanese-American men.[31] In this study, elevated SBP in midlife is associated with important endophenotypes such as low brain weight and greater amounts of neuritic plaque in the neocortex and hippocampus.[31] Also, elevated DBP related to greater numbers of neurofibrillary tangles in the hippocampus.[31] These findings support earlier observations by Sparks and colleagues[42] that increased blood pressure is associated with AD-related neuropathology in specific brain topologies central to the acquisition and storage of information.

Together, this evidence indicates that hypertension can directly increase dementia risk, and that the control of blood pressure can modify important endophenotypes and reduce dementia rates in persons with hypertension.

Nonrandomized Controlled Studies on the Relationship of Hypertension to Cognitive Loss

Given the array of cross-sectional and prospective data on the relationship of hypertension to cognitive loss, nonrandomized, controlled clinical studies are the next logical step. Few such studies have been completed, but many are underway.

Initial prospective studies focused primarily on treatment effects designed to normalize blood pressure without considerations for the class of medication used to achieve control, and most of them confirmed the beneficial effect as seen in the cross-sectional studies. For example, Guo and colleagues[43] showed that the use of antihypertensive treatment is associated with a significant reduction in the risk of cognitive loss in later years. To determine whether baseline hypertension and antihypertensive treatment predicts cognitive decline in elderly individuals, a fairly large longitudinal population-based study of 1373 elderly individuals was conducted in Nantes (western France). In this 4-year follow-up study, persons with hypertension who received treatment were compared with a control group, and the treatment group had lower cognitive decline at follow-up.[44] Another similarly designed study, but with a 5-year follow-up period of 1617 African Americans, observed a 38% reduction in cognitive decline in persons with hypertension treated with medication compared with untreated controls.[45] These prospective studies add an additional layer of evidence to cross-sectional studies to support the role of hypertension in the development of AD.

Building on evidence from the initial, less specific treatment studies, including those suggesting that calcium plays a key role in brain homeostasis leading to AD, Yasar and colleagues[46] investigated the relationship between the use of DHP- or non-DHP-CCBs with AD risk, using the Baltimore Longitudinal Study on Aging. From this study, an association between DHP-CCBs and reduced AD risk was observed, although not to a statistically significant level. In addition, the Cache County Study also showed that the use of potassium-sparing diuretic alone reduced the risk of AD by $\sim 47\%$, which is a relatively large effect.[47] Further, a 5-year follow-up study of a community sample of African Americans showed that antihypertensive and other medications affecting CVD risk factors is associated with $\sim 40\%$ reduction in the risk of incident dementia.[45] Using data from the Rotterdam study to examine the parallel relationship of hypertension to vascular dementia and AD, a significantly beneficial effect of treatment with medication is associated with performance on cognitive tasks, although a less-than-optimal effect on AD was reported.[48] Hanon and colleagues[49] showed a 42% reduction in the risk of developing AD in persons with hypertension receiving medication, a finding that is also supported by Khatchaturian and colleagues,[47] using a large population-based sample of 3308 persons from the Cache County cohort. These provided early evidence that maintenance of blood pressure in the normal range by medication is cognitively advantageous.

Inconsistency of the relationship of blood pressure to cognition in older adults led to the realization that treatment studies must also be attentive to the extent of blood pressure control. Whether an aggressive reduction in blood pressure can augment cognitive loss in the elderly became a concern of many in the field. To address this question, the Heart Outcomes Prevention Evaluation study prospectively evaluated the effects of medications to treat hypertension and showed that the greatest reduction in blood pressure is associated with enhanced cognitive function in demented elderly.[50] Conversely, few studies have documented a tendency for blood pressure to decrease in years immediately preceding dementia.[13,40,41] The implication of these conflicting observations is that unknown factors comediate the relationship of blood pressure treatment and control to cognitive dexterity.

Because AD is a chronic disease, potentially requiring years of insult for phenotypic expression to occur, much attention was given to whether or not the duration of uncontrolled hypertension contributes to the earlier inconsistencies of hypertension-related cognitive loss. To address this question, the Honolulu Aging Study recently examined the effects of the duration of treatment of hypertension on subsequent cognitive loss. From this study, Peila and colleagues[10] showed a 6% reduction in dementia risk for each additional year of treatment. Inherent in this finding is that the duration of treatment and control of hypertension, and perhaps the untreated and uncontrolled hypertension, are critical determinants of hypertension-related cognitive dexterity.

Collectively, these nonrandomized controlled trials add significantly to growing evidence that treatment of hypertension can delay or prevent associated cognitive loss; that blood pressure control is important; and that the duration of untreated and uncontrolled hypertension and the extent to which treatment and control are sustained play collective roles in the relationship between hypertension and cognitive dexterity. Importantly, these studies set the stage for randomized controlled trials and provide the momentum for a more detailed assessment of the differential class-effect of medication used to achieve blood pressure control.

Randomized Controlled Trials

Few large randomized controlled studies have added clarity to the relationship between the treatment and control of hypertension and future cognitive function as seen in the nonrandomized controlled studies. Although a few such studies failed to find significant differences between treatment groups, most reported that control of hypertension is beneficial to future cognitive stability.

Studies that reported a beneficial effect of treatment of hypertension not only added clarity, but also strengthened available evidence and the public health imperative for the treatment and control of hypertension. From the vascular dementia project,[18] a 2-year follow-up study of 2418 patients aged 60 and above with isolated systolic hypertension and randomized into treatment and control groups, a 50% reduction in hypertension-related cognitive loss was found in the treatment group. From the same study, an additional 2 years of follow-up after unbinding the sample showed that early intervention and the long-term treatment and control of hypertension can significantly reduce the risk of related cognitive deterioration as the population ages.[19] This observation, together with evidence from prospective but nonrandomized studies and from randomized but not placebo-controlled studies, supports the view that duration of untreated and/or uncontrolled hypertension is an important factor in the relationship between hypertension and future cognitive loss.

As evidence accumulated on the cognitively beneficial effects of treatment and control of hypertension, interest also grew on whether concomitant reduction in CVD risks and related phenotypes besides hypertension offers additional cognitive benefit. From the patient sample studied by Forette and colleagues,[18,19] a concomitant reduction in the rates of AD and vascular and mixed dementia was observed at 2- and 4-year follow-up points, suggesting that treatment and/or control of hypertension can also reduce AD and vascular– and mixed dementia–specific risks. Observation of 12% to 19% reduction in the risk of dementia and cognitive loss, respectively, in the Perindopril Protection Against Recurrent Stroke Study trial using perindopril (an ACE inhibitor) with or without indapamide in the treatment versus control groups[20] adds credence to earlier observations by Forette and colleagues.[18,19] Because hypertension in this sample was defined as an SBP of 160 mm Hg or higher and a DBP of 90 mm Hg or higher, treatment targets may have been insufficient for optimal cognitive benefits. These findings indicate that concomitant reduction in other CVD risk factors is incidental to the treatment of hypertension and may augment the benefits from hypertension treatment and/or control. Given that few other CVD risk factors are implicated as AD risk, it remains possible that reduction in these other risk factors can mechanistically explain the beneficial effects of treated but uncontrolled hypertension on cognition. As such, the HOPE trial, a randomized placebo-controlled study of 9297 patients with vascular disease or diabetes together with an additional CVD risk, followed up participants for an average of ∼4.5 years.[21] In this study, a significant 41% reduction in stroke-related cognitive decline was observed in the ACE inhibitor–treated group compared with the placebo group.

Conclusions from meta-analysis of the randomized placebo-controlled studies affirm the usefulness of treatment and control of hypertension in preventing future CVD- and AD-related cognitive decline in persons with hypertension.[51,52] In addition to blood pressure control, a concomitant improvement in other CVD risk markers during such treatment offers additional neuroprotection beyond what is provided by the control of blood pressure alone.

Negative results

Whereas most randomized controlled trials confirmed the idea that cognitive loss is associated with untreated hypertension, a few found no significant effect. For example, a 54-month follow-up study of 2584 older persons with hypertension treated with diuretics or β-blockers showed no difference between the treatment and control groups.[53] Building on the work of Prince and colleagues,[53] the Systolic Hypertension in the Elderly Program is a 5-year follow-up study that compared the incidence of dementia in a group of persons with hypertension treated with diuretics and/or β-blockers with placebo. Although the incidence of dementia tended to be lower in the treatment group, the difference did not reach statistical significance. Using ∼3.7-year follow-up data from the study on cognition and prognosis in the elderly, Lithell and colleagues[54] found no association between the groups of persons with hypertension treated with ARB and diuretic compared with controls. Also, while McGuinness and colleagues[55] showed ∼11% reduction in the risk of dementia in patients without earlier cerebral vascular accident (CVA), the difference was not significant. Also, the hypertension in the very elderly sub-study trial used a double-blind, placebo-controlled study to assess whether treatment of hypertension in patients aged 80 years and above would reduce the incidence of dementia, vascular dementia, and AD. Despite this tendency toward a beneficial effect, a nonsignificant hazard ratio of 0.86 was found in the study. Notably, the target blood pressure of 150 mm Hg SBP in the study may have been suboptimal for a cognitively beneficial effect of treatment.[22] For many of these negative studies, the extent to which the duration of exposure (for the untreated or the treated whose hypertension went uncontrolled) contributed to the cognitive outcome was not considered.

Whereas studies supporting the idea that the treatment and control of hypertension would be beneficial for minimizing future cognitive loss are hardly definitive, most of them reported a beneficial effect, and negative observations are in the minority. Together, they provide insight into the effects of blood pressure treatment and control on future cognitive function, and whether the choice of medication to treat elevated blood pressure is important to the cognitively beneficial effects.

Type of Antihypertensive Medication and Cognitive Benefit

Although conclusions from treatment studies indicate mostly beneficial effects, studies reporting negative results cannot be ignored. Explanations for negative findings have dwelled largely on study design, sample size, duration of exposure to hypertension, and the extent to which control with treatment was sustained. However, it is increasingly recognized that choice of antihypertensive medication may have differential cognitively beneficial effects. To address this question, the effect of medications affecting the posited mechanisms by which hypertension exerts its cognitively beneficial effects was recently examined. Such medications include mostly ACE inhibitors and ARBs. Medications such as CCBs considered to not favorably affect cognitive homeostasis were also examined.

Support for the cognitively beneficial effect of ACE inhibitors came from the work of Gard,[56] who demonstrated that ACE inhibitors have moderate effects on cognitive reserve, but that the ARB losartan has even significantly better beneficial effect on memory. Increasingly, white matter hyperintensity is observed to coexist with AD. Users of antihypertensive medications such as CCBs or loop diuretics have more severe white matter hyperintensity on MRI and worse performance on modified 3MS than users of β-blockers.[57] Together, the evidence indicates that ACE, and to a greater extent ARB, can augment the cognitively beneficial effect of blood pressure control in persons with hypertension.

Not all medications used to achieve control of blood pressure have cognitively beneficial effects. Building on the potential adverse cognitive effects associated with the use of CCBs in the elderly in cross-sectional studies, Maxwell and colleagues[58] examined prospectively the association of the use of CCBs and that of other antihypertensive drugs with cognition. From this study, the users of CCBs were significantly more likely than others to experience cognitive decline,[58] indicating that CCBs are associated with adverse cognitive outcomes. In an attempt to further crystallize the effects of the CCBs, Yasar and colleagues[46] showed that, although the DHP-CCBs tend to be beneficial, the non-DHP-CCBs actually propagate cognitive deterioration.

Collectively, these reports indicate that medications to treat hypertension have class effects—some exert beneficial effects; others do not. Antihypertensives having the ability to cross the blood-brain barrier and modify the renin-angiotensin-aldosterone system (such as perindopril or losartan) or brain calcium metabolism (nitrendipine) provide additional defense against cognitive loss beyond that provided by blood pressure control alone. Conversely, centrally acting sympatholytic agents and non-DHP-CCBs appear to promote cognitive loss. The beneficial effects of ARB suggest that angiotensin receptor ligands may have potential in the prevention or even reversal of dementias, specifically of the AD type.

SPECIAL CONSIDERATION ON THE ASSOCIATION OF HYPERTENSION WITH COGNITIVE FUNCTION
Low Blood Pressure and Memory Function

Although the investigation of the relationship of blood pressure to cognitive decline has focused largely on hypertension, the evidence also indicates that excessively low blood pressure can promote cognitive decline. Evidence from the NHANES III data suggests that low blood pressure exerts a negative cognitive consequence, especially in the very old (>80 years). Other published results assert increased incidence of dementia and AD in persons with low SBP or DBP, respectively. Because the duration of hypertension can modify blood pressure-related cognitive outcome, understanding of this relationship is critically important.[41,59,60] In addition to cross-sectional evidence, a few studies with sufficient follow-up time on the relationship of low blood pressure to cognitive decline are briefly discussed. From the Kungsholmen project, Qiu and colleagues[60] showed that low DBP (<70 mm Hg) in ~7 years before dementia diagnosis, while baseline evidence of cognitive function was controlled for, was associated with increased risk of dementia and AD. This finding was even stronger among those undergoing treatment for hypertension. Similarly, Qiu and colleagues[61] showed that a ≥15 mm Hg drop in SBP in subjects whose baseline SBP is less than 160 mm Hg predicted dementia and AD, especially in those suffering from vascular disorders such as CVA and diabetes. The 3-year follow-up data from the Gothenburg and Rotterdam studies also support the inverse association of SBP and DBP with dementia risk among those undergoing treatment for hypertension.[62] A long-duration follow-up study, the Bronx Aging Study on community-dwelling volunteers, showed that low DBP (<70 mm Hg) is associated with a nearly two-fold increase in dementia risk and AD. Persistently low DBP is associated with even greater risk of dementia and cognitive decline.[41]

Although the exact levels of cognitively beneficial blood pressure are yet to be quantified, a discussion of the effects of low blood pressure on cognition is incomplete without recognition of the age factor. Although treatments to lower blood pressure can enhance cognition, an aggressive reduction in blood pressure must be approached with caution, given the unanticipated negative cognitive consequences in the very old. Whether relatively low blood pressure is a complication of dementia of the AD type or whether it merely predisposes a subpopulation to an increased dementia risk needs further clarification.

Because chronic hypertension-induced endothelia-hyalinosis may compromise cerebral perfusion, maintenance of blood pressure in the optimal range in chronically hypertensive elderly may bring less than optimal benefit. It may further compromise adaptive physiologic mechanisms to enhance cerebral perfusion and combat cerebral oxygen deprivation in the very old. In addition to the considerations for comorbid conditions in the treatment of hypertension, the control of blood pressure in the very old must consider age and severity and duration of hypertension to optimize the benefits of such a treatment.

Pulse and Blood Pressure: Non-Linear Relationship to Cognitive Function

Similar to what was found in studies that examined the relationship of stages of hypertension to cognitive outcomes,[17] the relationship of PPR to cognitive reserve is predominantly nonlinear, and it is moderated by age and education. In addition to the evidence from the NHANES data, others have reported that low pulse and blood pressure can promote cognitive loss.[63,64] A significant association of PPR with increased AD risk was demonstrated in a Korean group, although with much smaller sample size than in the NHANES.[63] A finding not observed in the Korean study, but supported by published reports from Qiu and colleagues,[65] is a U-shaped relationship of PPR with cognitive performance. Higher and lower tertiles of PPR paralleled cognitive decline in a sample of 256 AD patients examined in this study. This finding is in concordance with results from Morris and colleagues[66] who reported a nonlinear relationship of hypertension with cognitive function using a biracial community sample. Also, from the Baltimore ongitudinal Study of Aging, Waldestein and colleagues[64] demonstrated a nonlinear relationship of hypertension with poor cognitive function. This evidence indicates that the relationship of PPR to cognitive dexterity is fairly complicated and nonlinear.

Similar to the relationship between PPR and cognitive performance, elevated blood pressure is nonlinearly related (U-shaped) to performance on cognitive tasks, especially in the old ($\geq$70 years). This effect is most significant in the very old (see **Fig. 4**). Although the exact understanding of this relationship needs further clarification, it is not known whether there is a threshold beyond which an increase in blood pressure can overcome the barrier to brain perfusion created by hypertension-induced endothelial dysfunction and cerebral autoregulatory mechanisms. Alternatively, selective CVD-related mortality in persons with severe hypertension offers a competing explanation. Collectively, this evidence suggests that hypertension is an important dementia risk factor, that the relationship between the two is nonlinear, and that it remains even after discounting the contribution of other important risk factors. Even if hypertension results in mild worsening of cognitive loss, and the early treatment and control of hypertension result in a slight reduction of dementia risk, the benefit of an early intervention can be substantial, given the high prevalence of hypertension and the growing magnitude of dementia as the United States population ages.

MECHANISM BY WHICH HYPERTENSION AFFECTS COGNITIVE FUNCTION
Overview

Although cerebral hypoperfusion and chronic oxygen deprivation appear central to the effects of hypertension on neurocognition and AD pathology, understanding of the exact mechanism mediating this relationship is a work in progress. Experimental investigations including animal studies provided the first line of evidence supporting several of the proposed mechanisms. Chronic hypertension-induced upregulation of vascular pathology appears to exert the most significant effects. For example, an important dementia precursor could be the unfavorable effects of hypertension on microvascular degeneration that alters cerebral endothelium. Second, hypertension-induced proliferation of smooth muscle cells, basal lamina alterations, luminal narrowing, endothelia-hyalinosis, and fibrosis have been reported to cause hypoperfusion and chronic cerebral oxygen insufficiency[67] and deranged glucose homeostasis such as in AD. Associated alteration in neurovascular coupling, complex autoregulatory system and consequent cerebral hypoperfusion often complicate these vascular changes. Third, the ACE, RAS, and nitric oxide (NO) pathways are central to the pathogenesis of hypertension and have been reported to mediate some of these vascular changes in persons with chronic hypertension. Also, direct independent effects of the ACE, RAS, and NO systems on neurocognition and AD pathology are increasingly recognized.

Endothelia-hyalinosis, reduced vascular compliance and fibrosis, neurovascular coupling, complex autoregulatory system, and cerebral hypoperfusion, independently or acting synergistically, appear to mediate the effects of chronic hypertension on neurocognition and AD pathology (**Fig. 6**). Indeed, these vascular changes may impair the ready flux of important biochemical and synaptic transmission. Alternatively, changes in the blood-brain barrier may result in increased vascular permeability, protein extravasations in the brain parenchyma, leading to amyloid β (Aβ)-protein accumulation.[68] It is also possible that independent but similar causal mechanisms may be responsible for hypertension and cognitive loss and AD pathology.

Hypertension and Cerebral Hypoperfusion

Cerebral perfusion and chronic cerebral oxygen insufficiency
Hypertension, cerebral hypoperfusion, and chronic cerebral oxygen insufficiency are causally linked to neurodegeneration. A complex, but delicate autoregulatory system

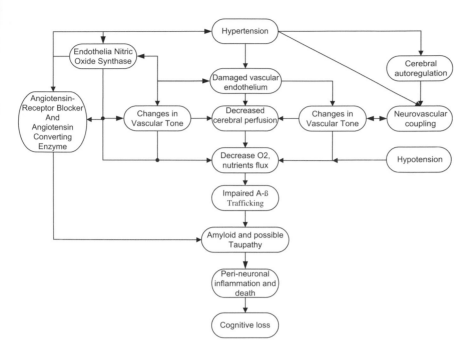

Note: Hypertension can cause direct damage to vascular endothelium and decrease cerebral perfusion. Hypertension-related alteration in cerebral autoregulatory mechanisms and neurovascular coupling can cause changes in vascular tone and reduce cerebral perfusion. Alternatively, direct hypertension-related damage to the endothelium may alter endothelia nitric oxide function with resultant change in vascular tone and cerebral hypoperfusion. Concomitant or hypertension-related changes in angiotensin receptor and or angiotensin converting enzyme can directly promote amyloid deposition as well as alter cerebral perfusion through changes in vascular tone. Below age-specific optimal blood pressure can directly reduce cerebral perfusion and promote chronic cerebral oxygen insufficiency, a common pathway by which hypertension-related β-amyloid pathology, peri-nueronal inflammation and consequent cognitive loss occurs.

Fig. 6. Mechanism by which hypertension affects cognitive function.

guides cerebral blood flow. Derangement of this autoregulatory system, such as imposed by hypertension, causes cerebral hypoperfusion and significantly alters neurotransmission essential to cognitive health. These changes, acting in concert with endothelial dysfunction in the small cerebral vessel, result in chronic cerebral oxygen deprivation and increased susceptibility to hypoxia.

The relevance of oxygen deprivation to proper neuronal and cognitive function was demonstrated by Lukiw and colleagues.[69] It was shown that in neural cell culture and in the hippocampus using in vivo models, cyclooxygenase-2 and presenile-1 are induced after only about 5 minutes of hypoxia.[69,70] From the available evidence, it is reasonable to conclude that cerebral hypoperfusion is an important common pathway by which vascular pathology exerts its deleterious effects on neurocognitive function. The ensuing discussion focuses on hypertension-related vascular derangements and their relationship to cerebral hypoperfusion.

Cerebral hypoperfusion and cognition
Results from studies in humans support a causal role for cerebral hypoperfusion in the pathogenesis of hypertension-related cognitive loss. Several of these studies also demonstrated a significant relationship between cerebral hypoperfusion and AD

phenotype.[71–73] Tsolaki and colleagues[74] reported that cerebral hypoperfusion is significantly associated with performance on the Cambridge Cognitive Examination. In support of the relationship between cerebral blood flow (CBF) and AD endophenotypes, Ueda[75] established that left posterior temporal regional CBF predicted performance on the clock drawing test. Independently, Jagust and colleagues,[76] Tsolaki and colleagues,[74] and Ushijima and colleagues[77] confirmed the link between performance on the mini mental state examination (MMSE) and hypoperfusion in the frontal, parietal, and temporal cortex. In the study by Ushijima and colleagues, attention and calculation showed a correlation with decline in CBF in the frontal cortex, whereas orientation and recall associated with attenuated CBF in posterior brain regions. Others have also reported on the relationship of CBF with AD endophenotypes and the rate of cognitive decline in AD. Nagahama and colleagues[78] showed that reduced CBF in the right posterodorsal, anterior, and superior prefrontal cortex and the inferior parietal cortex was most pronounced in the category of AD patients with rapidly progressing cognitive loss. It therefore appears that cerebral hypoperfusion has an etiologic role in the pathogenesis of AD.

In addition to the direct effect of hypertension, changes in PPR contribute to changes in cerebral hemodynamics. Increased PPR is a marker of increased arterial stiffness and widespread atherosclerosis,[79–81] both of which can cause cerebral hypoperfusion. Conversely, low PPR correlates with decreased blood ejection, low stroke volume, and decreased cerebral perfusion pressure. Because low and high PPR can cause cerebral hypoperfusion and chronic cerebral oxygen deprivation, they also likely contribute to hypertension-related cognitive loss.

Hypertension, Neurovascular Coupling, and Cognition

Hypertension-induced changes in neurovascular coupling have been suggested to associate with neurodegeneration. Such deranged processes may act through three important mechanisms: (1) changes in cerebrovascular function and structure, altering brain hypoperfusion; (2) alteration in vascular reactivity and activation of Aβ; and (3) other mechanisms yet to be fully characterized.

At the structural level, it is well established that cerebrovascular structures are significantly altered in AD.[82] Such alterations include reduction in the number of microvessels, flattening of endothelial cells, and degeneration of vascular smooth muscle.[82] In uncontrolled, long-standing hypertension, alteration in the vascular microcirculatory system results in neurovascular coupling and reduced brain perfusion. Such reduction in resting CBF has been suggested to attenuate the neuronal-related activation of compensatory increase in CBF.[83]

Newly emerging evidence suggests that hypertension-induced vascular changes can also directly promote Aβ pathology. Although in-depth understanding of this process is still evolving, it has been reported that by attenuating the activation of neuronal-related increase in compensatory CBF, neurovascular coupling directly upregulates Aβ formation. Significant dysregulation of cerebral circulation in mouse models of AD, mutated to overexpress APP and increase Aβ levels, supports the neurovascular coupling derangement hypothesis.[83] Also, attenuation of endothelia-dependent vascular response while reactions to vasoconstriction are exaggerated have also been found to exacerbate the upstream effects of hypertension-related dysregulation.[84,85] Presence of such alterations in vascular reactivity in isolated vessel of normal mouse exposed to Aβ$_{1-40}$[85,86] further supports the role of neurovascular coupling and strengthens the dysregulation hypothesis.

Other direct mechanisms may mediate the relationship of hypertension-related alteration in neurovascular coupling to AD. For example, vasoconstriction can alter the transfer of nutrients and oxygen supply to the brain. Less than optimal CBF may also alter Aβ trafficking across the blood-brain barrier[87] and reduce Aβ clearance while promoting its accumulation in the brain. Independently, reduced CBF may attenuate synthesis of protein central to optimal neuronal function and cognitive plasticity.

Changes in cerebrovascular function and structure and brain hypoperfusion, alteration in vascular reactivity and activation of Aβ, and other processes yet to be fully characterized are important mechanisms mediating the relationship of hypertension to cognitive health.

Hypertension, Cerebral Autoregulation, Hypometabolism, and Cognition

A distinct component of the cerebral autoregulatory system is linked to cerebral metabolism. During neuronal activity, an increase in oxygen usage is followed by immediate increase in CBF.[88] Such an increase in CBF maintains a near-constant oxygen and glucose delivery to the brain, therefore maintaining cerebral metabolism. Given this, an increase in oxygen and glucose uptake often indicates enhanced cerebral metabolism.[89] Because changes in cerebral metabolism can be deduced from regional cerebral perfusion, cerebral perfusion is used as an indicator of neuronal activity in neuroimaging studies.[83,90] An important protective system ensures near-constant CBF through autoregulation and prevents significant fluctuation in cerebral perfusion.[83,91,92] A compensatory, autoregulatory arterial-arteriolar bed dynamically adjusts the capacity and compliance of its vessels in response to changes in cerebral blood perfusion pressure (CPP) by dilating when CPP drops and constricting when CPP increases.[93] The ultimate goal of this process is to optimally deliver oxygen and glucose to brain tissue. In summary, hypertension can alter brain perfusion, impair oxygen and glucose delivery to the brain, and alter brain metabolism in AD.

Hypertension-related cerebromicrovascular pathology is central to the cerebral hypoperfusion in AD brain.[94–98] Similar to the effect of hypoperfusion on brain glucose homeostasis, a diminution in cerebral metabolism that results in decreased CBF can also exert negative cognitive effects.[99] Although consensus is lacking on whether reduced cerebral perfusion in AD brain precedes cerebral hypometabolism, given that years of hypertension and reduced cerebral perfusion are required for evident cognitive loss and cerebral hypometabolism,[98] it is reasonable to suggest that hypoperfusion in AD may also precede cerebral hypometabolism. In support of this view, Warkentin and colleagues[100] consistently observed diminution in cerebral glucose metabolism in the temporoparietal cortex of AD brain, whereas varying degrees of hypoperfusion were concomitantly observed in the frontal and occipital cortex of different AD patients. Late-onset AD patients demonstrating significant brain hypometabolism have attenuated perfusion in the hippocampal-amygdaloid complex, the anterior and posterior cingulate, and the anterior thalamus.[101,102] Regardless of the directionality of the association, collectively, the evidence mostly suggests that reduced CBF is linked to deranged cerebral glucose homeostasis, a hallmark of AD. Notably, significant evidence indicates that hypertension has an etiologic role in the development of cerebral hypoperfusion.

Hypertension, Brain Renin-Angiotensin System, Angiotensin-Converting Enzyme, and Cognition

Angiotensin II is a key factor in the pathogenesis of hypertension.[103] Also, the RAS system exerts a significant effect on cognitive function. Although this effect may be partly mediated through hypertension-related vascular dysfunction, available evidence also indicates that the RAS system can directly influence AD pathology in the brain. However, whether elevated blood pressure directly mediates RAS-related memory loss or RAS merely shares a common risk factor with hypertension and AD is yet to be ascertained. Nonetheless, the understanding of this relationship merits a brief discussion in this review.

More than 100 years have passed since the first component of the RAS, renin, isolated from the kidney extracts, was observed to induce vasopressor response in rabbits by Tiegerstedt in 1898. The RAS is a complex enzymatic pathway generating several active peptides that controls fluid homeostasis, blood pressure, hormone secretion, and behavioral and cognitive responses.[104,105] Although an active component of the RAS such as angiotensin II does not cross the blood-brain barrier, peripheral RAS can directly influence cerebral regions such as the circumventricular areas that lack the blood-brain barrier. Beyond the peripheral effects of RAS in such a brain region, an independent RAS also exists in the brain. The effects of RAS and ACE on the cognitive process are therefore exerted through several pathways: effects on blood pressure, direct effects on neurotrophic processes important to efficient learning and memory, direct effect on aggregation of Aβ, and effects on the cholinergic system.

Although evidence on the role of the RAS in learning and memory is contradictory, most studies support the view that angiotensin is harmful to cognitive processes.[106] The relationship of ACE to vascular disease and pathologies is one important way by which RAS exerts its effects on neurocognition.[107] The brain's RAS system regulates sympathetic activity and baroreflexes and contributes to neurogenic hypertension.[108] Higher ACE activity in plasma is closely associated with higher prevalence of hypertension, ischemic heart disease and lacuna strokes, and cognitive loss.[109] These associations indicate that a significant part of the effects of ACE on cognition may be mediated through its effects on blood pressure.

Although the RAS system may exert significant effect through its influence on blood pressure, much evidence also exists on additional, but direct and independent, effects on cognitive processes. In addition to its role in the modulation of blood pressure, RAS also exerts multiple additional functions in the brain, including processes of sensory information, learning, and memory.[106,110] Inhibitors of RAS, particularly ACE inhibitors and angiotensin II receptor antagonists, have been demonstrated to have potential neurotropic effects in various learning and memory paradigms.[111] Experimental studies also indicate that chronic long-term inhibition of the RAS can prevent most of the deleterious effects caused by aging in the cardiovascular system and the brain in normal mouse and rat.[112] Angiotensin II antagonist injection before and after a conditioned avoidance test facilitated learning and retention.[112,113] It acts directly on central RAS receptors to enhance associative memory and learning, possibly with a differential effect on acquisition, storage, and recall.[113] In support of earlier findings, Gard and colleagues[106] demonstrated that ACE inhibitors have cognitive enhancing effects, and they enhance learning in rats. This evidence supports the view that the RAS system, which is central to the pathogenesis of hypertension, may also have an additional but important role in cognitive processing that is independent of its effects on blood pressure.

At the molecular levels, and independent of hypertension effect, RAS directly promotes aggregation, deposition, and fibril formation of neurotoxic Aβ in the AD brain.[114] If RAS were a promoter of AD pathology, an opposing effect would be expected with ACE inhibitor. Indeed, ACE inhibitors directly reduce Aβ aggregation, attenuate Aβ fibril formation, and prevent neuronal cell death from Aβ-induced neurotoxicity, ultimately reducing susceptibility to AD.[114] These indicate that RAS can directly promote Aβ formation, and that this effect is attenuated by ACE inhibitor.

The cholinergic system is involved in cognitive processes. A direct link of RAS and ACE to the cholinergic system has also been established. Because angiotensin II can have an inhibitory effect on acetylcholine release, it is believed that inhibitors of this biochemical process, such as ACE inhibitors, can enhance cognition through the release of acetylcholine. Supporting this view, Denny and colleagues[115] showed that angiotensin II blocked long-term potentiation in the hippocampus and amygdala. Therefore, angiotensin II receptor blockers would be expected to have effects on cognitive processes that are similar to those of ACE inhibitors. It is recommended that future studies on the relationship of angiotensin II remain cognizant of its complex relationship with learning so that they do not misinterpret any apparent inconsistencies that show an inhibitory action at low doses but an enhancing effect at higher doses. Failure to recognize such differential relationships may slow scientific advancement in the understanding of this relationship.[116]

Hypertension, Endothelial NO, and Cognitive Function

Dysfunctionality of NO metabolism is central to the pathogenesis of hypertension and cerebral hypoperfusion that occurs in AD.[117] Nitric oxide contributes to the functional vascular changes under pathologic conditions, such as those observed in hypertension.[118] Nitric oxide derived from vascular eNOS is involved in vascular tone, blood pressure modulation, vascular homeostasis, and ultimately cerebral perfusion. Because cerebral autoregulation is mediated by NO, an efficient eNOS system attenuates atherosclerosis and thrombosis and improves blood flow by lowering stress on the blood vessel walls. By doing so, NO protects the endothelial cell function, which is an important mediator of hypertension-related vascular dysregulation and dysfunctionality.[119]

Longstanding, untreated, and uncontrolled hypertension acting in concert with the NO system results in cerebral hypoperfusion. Through the disturbance of basal NO levels, chronic hypertension causes alteration in the endothelium and induces vascular injury.[120] As cerebral perfusion decreases below a certain critical point, eNOS attempts to maintain vascular homeostasis by upregulating NO.[94–97] When this attempt fails, NO deregulation ensues. Together with hypoperfusion, the resulting damage to the endothelium impairs glucose flux to the brain,[121] a process that heralds the development of cognitive loss. Independent of hypoperfusion-related dysfunctionality of the NO system, hypertension-related deterioration in NO homeostasis and associated oxidative alterations also directly contributes to neuronal cell death, such as that seen in AD.[122–124]

Evidence is also growing to suggest that hypertension-related dysfunction in the NO system acts synergistically with the cholinergic receptors to directly promote AD pathology. In conscious rat, Nakajima and colleagues[126] showed that the activation of nicotinic acetylcholine receptors with consequent neural vasodilatation contributes to an increase in CBF and NO production in the hippocampus.[125,126] Implicit in this finding is that basal forebrain and medial septal cholinergic neurons may have direct projections onto the eNOS-positive interneuron with the possibility of important access to vasodilatation mechanism through the release of NO. Evidently, the entire cortical system, including the hippocampus, is densely innervated by a fine network of eNOS-positive fibers, which derived its origin from scattered eNOS-positive interneuron. The study by Moro and colleagues,[127] which supports the inference from the work of Nakajima and colleagues,[126] demonstrates the colocalization of NOS and muscarinic receptors in interneurons in neocortical regions projecting onto cerebral microvessels. Cholinergic denervation of NOS expressing interneurons and cortical microvessels is present especially in the temporal cortex of AD patients.[128,129] Collectively, these observations indicate that the basal forebrain cholinergic system has important effects on cortical blood flow regulation. Such changes in CBF are mediated by NO production through NOS interneurons provided by the nicotinic and muscarinic postsynaptic receptor system. Dysregulation of this system by chronic hypertension may be another important mechanism by which hypertension exerts its effects on cognitive processes.

Hypertension, Genetics, and Cognition

Contribution of genetic risk factors to disease phenotypes has been long established. Scientific advances during the last decade indicate that most such factors are not deterministic but instead act in concert with other environmental influences. A few such gene variants are now considered to have pleiotropic properties, allowing them to influence more than one pathologic process. Two such phenotypes are hypertension and neurocognitive loss. Although a complete discussion of the pleiotropic effects of such genetic variants influencing hypertension and cognitive loss is not possible in this review, the pleiotropic effects of variations at the ApoE and ACE loci are briefly discussed.

Genetic variation at the apolipoprotein e locus and cerebral hypoperfusion

Hypertension is causally linked to cerebral hypoperfusion. Evidence that a genetic variant potentiates cerebral hypoperfusion from a variety of causes is also known. The apolipoprotein E4 allele of the APOE *gene* (ApoE4) is the most consistent nondeterministic genetic risk factor for sporadic AD. Although several mechanisms are currently proposed to explain its effect on cognitive health, its relationship to cerebral hypoperfusion is increasingly noted, given the susceptibility of CBF to variation at the APOE locus. For example, ApoE4 associates with decrease in CBF velocity and enhances cerebrovascular amyloidogenesis in AD.[130] It also associates with reduction in CBF in the parietal, temporal, and occipital areas in AD. However, whether ApoE4 directly potentiates the hypertension-related hypoperfusion resulting in decreased cerebral metabolism is yet to be established.

Genetic variation at the ACE locus and cognition

The vasoconstriction property of ACE is central to the pathogenesis of hypertension.Variations at the ACE *gene* locus have been associated with increased AD risk. Consistently, polymorphism in which there is deletion rather than insertion of a 287-base-pair sequence in intron 16 of the human ACE *gene* has been associated with increased serum ACE activity and therefore elevation of blood pressure.[131] In humans homozygous for the D allele of the ACE *gene*, circulating ACE levels were found to be twice as high. However, studies on the relationship of ACE and AD have reported conflicting results. In a cohort of 350 AD patients, ACE I allele frequency was 28%, whereas another study found similar frequency in AD patients and Parkinson disease coexisting with AD pathology.[132] A few other studies failed to confirm such an association,[133,134] but instead observed an increase in ACE D allele prevalence and a reduced ACE I allele prevalence in older adults with age-associated memory loss.[135] In a 4-year longitudinal study of 1168 subjects to investigate cognitive decline in older adults with different I/D genotypes, a strong association of homozygous ACE DD allele with lower performance on cognitive measures compared with subjects with ID and II alleles was reported.[136] Although it seems premature to conclusively consider ACE *gene* polymorphism as a marker for AD, the pleiotropic effect of ACE on hypertension, as well as on memory decline and/or AD, must be considered. Nonetheless, its effects on vasoconstriction, elevated blood pressure, and consequent cerebral hypoperfusion and cognitive loss are increasingly recognized.

PREVENTION

Preservation of neurocognitive function among those showing earliest signs and symptoms of AD ameliorates the physical, emotional, and economic burden associated with the disease. Unfortunately, this benefit and the national goals of Healthy People 2010 cannot be realized without an efficient AD prevention strategy. Although medical treatment after disease onset may reduce disease progression and mortality, eventually, increases in disease prevalence will substantially escalate total disease burden in the population. Whereas the current approach to symptomatic treatment of AD may not be cost-effective in populations with excessive rates of disease (such as African Americans), an intervention strategy with dual applicability for primary and secondary prevention is likely to be more beneficial.

Given the increases in the rates of hypertension and memory disorder with advancing age and the relationships of hyper- and hypotension with cognitive loss, available evidence indicates that aggressive control of elevated blood pressure to prevent dementia in the very old is unlikely to be an efficient public health goal. For hypertension to cofactor the initiation of neurodegeneration, more than 1 to 1.5 decades of uncontrolled hypertension may be required (see **Fig. 5**). These intervals vary depending on whether or not blood pressure is treated and controlled or uncontrolled. An additional 2 decades may be needed from the initiation of neurodegeneration to the phenotypic expression of meaningful cognitive loss. Cumulatively, from the onset of hypertension to the appearance of clinically significant cognitive loss, an interval of ~35 years may be required for hypertension to result in dementia. The actual duration is subject to the presence of other risk factors or lack of them. Therefore, for public health intervention to have a maximal impact, such efforts must be directed at preventing or aggressively controlling hypertension at the earliest possible stage, before the establishment of arterial stiffness and the need for higher pressure for optimal cerebral perfusion. Using JNC VII criteria, cognitively beneficial target blood pressure should be in the normal range (<120/80 mm Hg) for persons aged less than 75; for persons aged 75 or older who have new-onset hypertension; and for diabetics irrespective of age. For persons aged 75 or older who have chronic hypertension, blood pressure in the prehypertensive range (120–139 mm Hg) is likely to be cognitively beneficial. Regardless of the duration and history of hypertension, cognitively beneficial target blood pressure for persons aged 80 or older should also remain in the prehypertensive range.

LIMITATIONS OF THE CURRENT KNOWLEDGE

Although most studies on the relationship of blood pressure to cognitive function reported beneficial effects of blood pressure in the normal range, a few found no relationship of elevated blood pressure with enhanced cognitive function. Others reported relationships ranging from a J- to a U-shape. Because this is newly emerging evidence, most of these studies were population-based, often involving large numbers of subjects. Mostly, the studies varied in their inclusion and exclusion criteria and in their classification of hypertension, including the range of blood pressure that was considered normal. Because they are mostly nonprospective in nature, the investigators were constrained by the cognitive measure originally used in these studies. Given the multitude of neuropsychological measures to choose from, it is not surprising that many of these studies used different cognitive batteries to assess different cognitive domains. Because the exact cognitive domain that is mostly affected by hypertension is yet to be ascertained, it not surprising that the results from these studies were varied.

It should be emphasized that cross-sectional studies are limited in their ability to establish directionality, because blood pressure and cognitive outcomes are assessed simultaneously. Because prospective studies have the advantage of time, measuring exposure to blood pressure and cognitive outcomes later on in life, it is rational to expect that they would be advantageous in assessing the association between blood pressure and cognitive reserve. Although most studies have demonstrated an association between elevated blood pressure and cognitive loss, there remains inconsistency in the findings. Possible explanations for this inconsistency include differences in sample size, duration of follow-up, and inclusion–exclusion criteria; the extent to which subjects' blood pressures were controlled; duration of medication use; and the type of psychological measures and cognitive domains that were assessed. Whether or not important covariants such as age, gender, ethnicity, education, aerobic fitness, body mass index, type 2 diabetes, and genetic variations at the APOE locus were considered may have contributed to such inconsistencies.

For the available randomized controlled trials, cognition was not the primary endpoint for most, which calls into question the design of such studies.It appears that certain classes or particular medications are more cognitively beneficial than others. Classes of medication used in most of the available randomized studies varied, ranging from diuretics, β-blockers, non-DHP- and DHP-CCBs, ACE inhibitors, and ARBs. In spite of the evidence that showed that the duration of treatment is important to the cognitively beneficial treatment effects, often, treatment duration was either not considered or not reported in most of these studies. Finally, it appears that long duration of hypertension may be required for its harmful effects on cognitive outcomes to manifest. Because cognitive outcomes were not the primary endpoint for most of these studies, they were unlikely to be of sufficient duration or of adequate power, or they used alternative approaches such as an enriched sample to compensate for duration and power to detect differences.

Because the NHANES III data are some of the most important data available on the national estimates of the prevalence of hypertension and its relationship to cognitive function, their limitations are worth special consideration. The NHANES III is advantaged in that it permits age-stratified analysis and adjustment for multiple confounders and therefore is a more robust assessment of the relationship of blood pressure and PPR to cognitive measure. Several unavoidable limitations of the NHANES data include possible bias from survey nonresponse and from missing values for some variables, and bias from self-reported history of hypertension as in other cross-sectional studies. Fortunately, the conclusions by Obisesan and colleagues[17] are not based on self-reported hypertension but rather on actual blood pressure measurements.

SUMMARY

Cumulative evidence implicates hypertension in the pathogenesis of AD. Although it may not presently be possible to completely discern the effects of treatment and control of hypertension itself from that of the medication used to achieve such treatment goals, efforts directed at the treatment and control of hypertension have significant public health impact.

Public health goals for optimal blood pressure should probably be age-specific. Because optimal blood pressure for optimal cognitive performance is yet to be clearly established and the undesirable effect of excessive reduction in blood pressure is not fully understood, the following recommendations are made using JNC VII criteria: target blood pressure beneficial to cognition should be in the normal range (<120/

80 mm Hg) for persons 75 years or younger, for persons aged 75 or older having new-onset hypertension, and for persons with diabetes irrespective of age. For persons aged 75 or older who have chronic hypertension, blood pressure in the prehypertensive range (120–139 mm Hg) is likely to be cognitively beneficial. Regardless of duration and history of hypertension, cognitively beneficial target blood pressure for persons aged 80 or older should also remain in the prehypertensive range.

If indeed hypertension is a risk factor for AD or shares the same pathophysiology, it is logical to expect that measures directed at blood pressure control will enhance cognitive reserve. This is an important public health goal.

REFERENCES

1. Johnson P. Fiscal implications of population ageing. Philos Trans R Soc Lond B Biol Sci 1997;352:1895–903.
2. Serow WJ. Economic and fiscal implications of aging for subnational American governments. J Aging Soc Policy 2001;12:47–63.
3. Covinsky KE, Eng C, Lui LY, et al. The last 2 years of life: functional trajectories of frail older people. J Am Geriatr Soc 2003;51:492–8.
4. Hamel E, Nicolakakis N, Aboulkassim T, et al. Oxidative stress and cerebrovascular dysfunction in mouse models of Alzheimer's disease. Exp Physiol 2008;93: 116–20.
5. Breteler MM, van den Ouweland FA, Grobbee DE, et al. A community-based study of dementia: the Rotterdam Elderly Study. Neuroepidemiology 1992; 11(Suppl 1):23–8.
6. Hachinski V, Munoz DG. Cerebrovascular pathology in Alzheimer's disease: cause, effect or epiphenomenon? Ann N Y Acad Sci 1997;826:1–6.
7. White L, Petrovitch H, Hardman J, et al. Cerebrovascular pathology and dementia in autopsied Honolulu-Asia aging study participants. Ann N Y Acad Sci 2002;977:9–23.
8. Van Nostrand WE, Davis-Salinas J, Saporito-Irwin SM. Amyloid beta-protein induces the cerebrovascular cellular pathology of Alzheimer's disease and related disorders. Ann N Y Acad Sci 1996;777:297–302.
9. Tzourio C. Hypertension, cognitive decline, and dementia: an epidemiological perspective. Dialogues Clin Neurosci 2007;9:61–70.
10. Peila R, White LR, Masaki K, et al. Reducing the risk of dementia: efficacy of long-term treatment of hypertension. Stroke 2006;37:1165–70.
11. Kivipelto M, Helkala EL, Hanninen T, et al. Midlife vascular risk factors and late-life mild cognitive impairment: a population-based study. Neurology 2001;56: 1683–9.
12. Launer LJ, Ross GW, Petrovitch H, et al. Midlife blood pressure and dementia: the Honolulu-Asia aging study. Neurobiol Aging 2000;21:49–55.
13. Skoog I, Lernfelt B, Landahl S, et al. 15-year longitudinal study of blood pressure and dementia. Lancet 1996;347:1141–5.
14. Frishman WH. Are antihypertensive agents protective against dementia? A review of clinical and preclinical data. Heart Dis 2002;4:380–6.
15. Manolio TA, Olson J, Longstreth WT. Hypertension and cognitive function: pathophysiologic effects of hypertension on the brain. Curr Hypertens Rep 2003;5: 255–61.
16. Korf ES, White LR, Scheltens P, et al. Midlife blood pressure and the risk of hippocampal atrophy: the Honolulu Asia aging study. Hypertension 2004;44:29–34.

17. Obisesan TO, Obisesan OA, Martins S, et al. High blood pressure, hypertension, and high pulse pressure are associated with poorer cognitive function in persons aged 60 and older: the Third National Health and Nutrition Examination Survey. J Am Geriatr Soc 2008;56:501–9.

18. Forette F, Seux ML, Staessen JA, et al. Prevention of dementia in randomised double-blind placebo-controlled Systolic Hypertension in Europe (Syst-Eur) trial. Lancet 1998;352:1347–51.

19. Forette F, Seux ML, Staessen JA, et al. The prevention of dementia with antihypertensive treatment: new evidence from the Systolic Hypertension in Europe (Syst-Eur) study. Arch Intern Med 2002;162:2046–52.

20. Tzourio C, Anderson C, Chapman N, et al. Effects of blood pressure lowering with perindopril and indapamide therapy on dementia and cognitive decline in patients with cerebrovascular disease. Arch Intern Med 2003;163:1069–75.

21. Bosch J, Yusuf S, Pogue J, et al. Use of ramipril in preventing stroke: double blind randomised trial. BMJ 2002;324:699–702.

22. Peters R, Beckett N, Forette F, et al. Incident dementia and blood pressure lowering in the Hypertension in the Very Elderly Trial cognitive function assessment (HYVET-COG): a double-blind, placebo controlled trial. Lancet Neurol 2008;7:683–9.

23. Kahonen-Vare M, Brunni-Hakala S, Lindroos M, et al. Left ventricular hypertrophy and blood pressure as predictors of cognitive decline in old age. Aging Clin Exp Res 2004;16:147–52.

24. Kuo HK, Sorond F, Iloputaife I, et al. Effect of blood pressure on cognitive functions in elderly persons. J Gerontol A Biol Sci Med Sci 2004;59:1191–4.

25. Waldstein SR, Brown JR, Maier KJ, et al. Diagnosis of hypertension and high blood pressure levels negatively affect cognitive function in older adults. Ann Behav Med 2005;29:174–80.

26. Waldstein SR, Katzel LI. Stress-induced blood pressure reactivity and cognitive function. Neurology 2005;64:1746–9.

27. The sixth report of the Joint National Committee on prevention, detection, evaluation, and treatment of high blood pressure. Arch Intern Med 1997;157:2413–46.

28. St Clair D, Whalley LJ. Hypertension, multi-infarct dementia and Alzheimer's disease. Br J Psychiatry 1983;143:274–6.

29. Sadowski M, Pankiewicz J, Scholtzova H, et al. Links between the pathology of Alzheimer's disease and vascular dementia. Neurochem Res 2004;29:1257–66.

30. Reitz C, Patel B, Tang MX, et al. Relation between vascular risk factors and neuropsychological test performance among elderly persons with Alzheimer's disease. J Neurol Sci 2007;257:194–201.

31. Petrovitch H, Ross GW, Steinhorn SC, et al. AD lesions and infarcts in demented and non-demented Japanese-American men. Ann Neurol 2005;57:98–103.

32. Petrovitch H, White LR, Izmirilian G, et al. Midlife blood pressure and neuritic plaques, neurofibrillary tangles, and brain weight at death: the HAAS. Honolulu-Asia aging study. Neurobiol Aging 2000;21:57–62.

33. Cacciatore F, Abete P, Ferrara N, et al. The role of blood pressure in cognitive impairment in an elderly population. Osservatorio Geriatrico Campano Group. J Hypertens 1997;15:135–42.

34. Richards SS, Emsley CL, Roberts J, et al. The association between vascular risk factor-mediating medications and cognition and dementia diagnosis in a community-based sample of African-Americans. J Am Geriatr Soc 2000;48:1035–41.

35. Hajjar I, Catoe H, Sixta S, et al. Cross-sectional and longitudinal association between antihypertensive medications and cognitive impairment in an elderly population. J Gerontol A Biol Sci Med Sci 2005;60:67–73.
36. Lindsay J, Laurin D, Verreault R, et al. Risk factors for Alzheimer's disease: a prospective analysis from the Canadian study of health and aging. Am J Epidemiol 2002;156:445–53.
37. Morris MS, Jacques PF, Rosenberg IH, et al. Hyperhomocysteinemia associated with poor recall in the third National Health and Nutrition Examination Survey. Am J Clin Nutr 2001;73:927–33.
38. Duron E, Hanon O. Vascular risk factors, cognitive decline, and dementia. Vasc Health Risk Manag 2008;4:363–81.
39. Bellew KM, Pigeon JG, Stang PE, et al. Hypertension and the rate of cognitive decline in patients with dementia of the Alzheimer type. Alzheimer Dis Assoc Disord 2004;18:208–13.
40. Hanon O, Haulon S, Lenoir H, et al. Relationship between arterial stiffness and cognitive function in elderly subjects with complaints of memory loss. Stroke 2005;36:2193–7.
41. Verghese J, Lipton RB, Hall CB, et al. Low blood pressure and the risk of dementia in very old individuals. Neurology 2003;61:1667–72.
42. Sparks DL, Scheff SW, Liu H, et al. Increased incidence of neurofibrillary tangles (NFT) in non-demented individuals with hypertension. J Neurol Sci 1995;131: 162–9.
43. Guo Z, Viitanen M, Winblad B, et al. Low blood pressure and incidence of dementia in a very old sample: dependent on initial cognition. J Am Geriatr Soc 1999;47:723–6.
44. Tzourio C, Dufouil C, Ducimetiere P, et al. Cognitive decline in individuals with high blood pressure: a longitudinal study in the elderly. EVA Study Group. Epidemiology of Vascular Aging. Neurology 1999;53:1948–52.
45. Murray MD, Lane KA, Gao S, et al. Preservation of cognitive function with antihypertensive medications: a longitudinal analysis of a community-based sample of African Americans. Arch Intern Med 2002;162:2090–6.
46. Yasar S, Corrada M, Brookmeyer R, et al. Calcium channel blockers and risk of AD: the Baltimore longitudinal study of aging. Neurobiol Aging 2005;26: 157–63.
47. Khachaturian AS, Zandi PP, Lyketsos CG, et al. Antihypertensive medication use and incident Alzheimer disease: the Cache County Study. Arch Neurol 2006;63: 686–92.
48. Salas M, In't Veld BA, van der Linden PD, et al. Impaired cognitive function and compliance with antihypertensive drugs in elderly: the Rotterdam Study. Clin Pharmacol Ther 2001;70:561–6.
49. Hanon O, Pequignot R, Seux ML, et al. Relationship between antihypertensive drug therapy and cognitive function in elderly hypertensive patients with memory complaints. J Hypertens 2006;24:2101–7.
50. Starr JM, Whalley LJ, Deary IJ. The effects of antihypertensive treatment on cognitive function: results from the HOPE study. J Am Geriatr Soc 1996;44: 411–5.
51. Feigin V, Ratnasabapathy Y, Anderson C. Does blood pressure lowering treatment prevent dementia or cognitive decline in patients with cardiovascular and cerebrovascular disease? J Neurol Sci 2005;229-230:151–5.
52. Birkenhager WH, Staessen JA. Progress in cardiovascular diseases: cognitive function in essential hypertension. Prog Cardiovasc Dis 2006;49:1–10.

53. Prince MJ, Bird AS, Blizard RA, et al. Is the cognitive function of older patients affected by antihypertensive treatment? Results from 54 months of the Medical Research Council's trial of hypertension in older adults. BMJ 1996;312:801–5.
54. Lithell H, Hansson L, Skoog I, et al. The Study on Cognition and Prognosis in the Elderly (SCOPE): principal results of a randomized double-blind intervention trial. J Hypertens 2003;21:875–86.
55. McGuinness B, Todd S, Passmore P, et al. The effects of blood pressure lowering on development of cognitive impairment and dementia in patients without apparent prior cerebrovascular disease. Cochrane Database Syst Rev 2006;2:CD004034.
56. Gard PR. Angiotensin as a target for the treatment of Alzheimer's disease, anxiety and depression. Expert Opin Ther Targets 2004;8:7–14.
57. Heckbert SR, Longstreth WT Jr, Psaty BM, et al. The association of antihypertensive agents with MRI white matter findings and with modified mini-mental state examination in older adults. J Am Geriatr Soc 1997;45:1423–33.
58. Maxwell CJ, Hogan DB, Ebly EM. Calcium-channel blockers and cognitive function in elderly people: results from the Canadian study of health and aging. CMAJ 1999;161:501–6.
59. Morris MC, Scherr PA, Hebert LE, et al. Association of incident Alzheimer disease and blood pressure measured from 13 years before to 2 years after diagnosis in a large community study. Arch Neurol 2001;58:1640–6.
60. Qiu C, von Strauss E, Fastbom J, et al. Low blood pressure and risk of dementia in the Kungsholmen project: a 6-year follow-up study. Arch Neurol 2003;60:223–8.
61. Qiu C, von Strauss E, Winblad B, et al. Decline in blood pressure over time and risk of dementia: a longitudinal study from the Kungsholmen project. Stroke 2004;35:1810–5.
62. Ruitenberg A, Skoog I, Ott A, et al. Blood pressure and risk of dementia: results from the Rotterdam study and the Gothenburg H-70 Study. Dement Geriatr Cogn Disord 2001;12:33–9.
63. Lee AY, Jeong SH, Choi BH, et al. Pulse pressure correlates with leukoaraiosis in Alzheimer disease. Arch Gerontol Geriatr 2006;42:157–66.
64. Waldstein SR, Giggey PP, Thayer JF, et al. Nonlinear relations of blood pressure to cognitive function: the Baltimore Longitudinal Study of Aging. Hypertension 2005;45:374–9.
65. Qiu C, Winblad B, Viitanen M, et al. Pulse pressure and risk of Alzheimer disease in persons aged 75 years and older: a community-based, longitudinal study. Stroke 2003;34:594–9.
66. Morris MC, Scherr PA, Hebert LE, et al. Association between blood pressure and cognitive function in a biracial community population of older persons. Neuroepidemiology 2002;21:123–30.
67. Perlmutter LS, Barron E, Saperia D, et al. Association between vascular basement membrane components and the lesions of Alzheimer's disease. J Neurosci Res 1991;30:673–81.
68. Hardy JA, Mann DM, Wester P, et al. An integrative hypothesis concerning the pathogenesis and progression of Alzheimer's disease. Neurobiol Aging 1986; 7:489–502.
69. Lukiw WJ, Bazan NG. Cyclooxygenase 2 RNA message abundance, stability, and hypervariability in sporadic Alzheimer neocortex. J Neurosci Res 1997;50:937–45.
70. Perkins DJ, Kniss DA. Tumor necrosis factor-alpha promotes sustained cyclooxygenase-2 expression: attenuation by dexamethasone and NSAIDs. Prostaglandins 1997;54:727–43.

71. Modzelewski R, de la Rue T, Janvresse E, et al. Development and validation of the random walk algorithm: application to the classification of diffuse heterogeneity in brain SPECT perfusion images. J Comput Assist Tomogr 2008;32:651–9.
72. Waragai M, Mizumura S, Yamada T, et al. Differentiation of early-stage Alzheimer's disease from other types of dementia using brain perfusion single photon emission computed tomography with easy Z-score imaging system analysis. Dement Geriatr Cogn Disord 2008;26:547–55.
73. Kobayashi S, Tateno M, Utsumi K, et al. Quantitative analysis of brain perfusion SPECT in Alzheimer's disease using a fully automated regional cerebral blood flow quantification software, 3DSRT. J Neurol Sci 2008;264:27–33.
74. Tsolaki M, Sakka V, Gerasimou G, et al. Correlation of rCBF (SPECT), CSF tau, and cognitive function in patients with dementia of the Alzheimer's type, other types of dementia, and control subjects. Am J Alzheimers Dis Other Demen 2001;16:21–31.
75. Ueda H, Kitabayashi Y, Narumoto J, et al. Relationship between clock drawing test performance and regional cerebral blood flow in Alzheimer's disease: a single photon emission computed tomography study. Psychiatry Clin Neurosci 2002;56(1):25–9.
76. Jagust WJ, Eberling JL, Reed BR, et al. Clinical studies of cerebral blood flow in Alzheimer's disease. Ann N Y Acad Sci 1997;826:254–62.
77. Ushijima Y, Okuyama C, Mori S, et al. Relationship between cognitive function and regional cerebral blood flow in Alzheimer's disease. Nucl Med Commun 2002;23:779–84.
78. Nagahama Y, Nabatame H, Okina T, et al. Cerebral correlates of the progression rate of the cognitive decline in probable Alzheimer's disease. Eur Neurol 2003; 50:1–9.
79. Bots ML, Witteman JC, Hofman A, et al. Low diastolic blood pressure and atherosclerosis in elderly subjects. The Rotterdam study. Arch Intern Med 1996;156:843–8.
80. Liao D, Arnett DK, Tyroler HA, et al. Arterial stiffness and the development of hypertension. The ARIC study. Hypertension 1999;34:201–6.
81. Chambless LE, Folsom AR, Davis V, et al. Risk factors for progression of common carotid atherosclerosis: the Atherosclerosis Risk in Communities Study, 1987–1998. Am J Epidemiol 2002;155:38–47.
82. Farkas E, Luiten PG. Cerebral microvascular pathology in aging and Alzheimer's disease. Prog Neurobiol 2001;64:575–611.
83. Iadecola C. Neurovascular regulation in the normal brain and in Alzheimer's disease. Nat Rev Neurosci 2004;5:347–60.
84. Iadecola C, Zhang F, Niwa K, et al. SOD1 rescues cerebral endothelial dysfunction in mice overexpressing amyloid precursor protein. Nat Neurosci 1999;2:157–61.
85. Niwa K, Porter VA, Kazama K, et al. A beta-peptides enhance vasoconstriction in cerebral circulation. Am J Physiol Heart Circ Physiol 2001;281:H2417–24.
86. Crawford F, Suo Z, Fang C, et al. Characteristics of the in vitro vasoactivity of beta-amyloid peptides. Exp Neurol 1998;150:159–68.
87. Zlokovic BV, Deane R, Sallstrom J, et al. Neurovascular pathways and Alzheimer amyloid beta-peptide. Brain Pathol 2005;15:78–83.
88. Attwell D, Iadecola C. The neural basis of functional brain imaging signals. Trends Neurosci 2002;25:621–5.
89. Ide K, Secher NH. Cerebral blood flow and metabolism during exercise. Prog Neurobiol 2000;61:397–414.

90. Wolf RL, Alsop DC, Levy-Reis I, et al. Detection of mesial temporal lobe hypoperfusion in patients with temporal lobe epilepsy by use of arterial spin labeled perfusion MR imaging. AJNR Am J Neuroradiol 2001;22:1334–41.

91. Heistad DD. Summary of symposium on cerebral blood flow: effect of nerves and neurotransmitters. Cardiovascular Center, University of Iowa, Iowa City, Iowa, June 16–18, 1981. J Cereb Blood Flow Metab 1981;1:447–50.

92. Baumbach GL, Heistad DD. Regional, segmental, and temporal heterogeneity of cerebral vascular autoregulation. Ann Biomed Eng 1985;13:303–10.

93. Daley ML, Pourcyrous M, Timmons SD, et al. Assessment of cerebrovascular autoregulation: changes of highest modal frequency of cerebrovascular pressure transmission with cerebral perfusion pressure. Stroke 2004;35:1952–6.

94. de la Torre JC. Critical threshold cerebral hypoperfusion causes Alzheimer's disease? Acta Neuropathol 1999;98:1–8.

95. de la Torre JC. Impaired cerebromicrovascular perfusion. Summary of evidence in support of its causality in Alzheimer's disease. Ann N Y Acad Sci 2000;924: 136–52.

96. de la Torre JC. Critically attained threshold of cerebral hypoperfusion: the CATCH hypothesis of Alzheimer's pathogenesis. Neurobiol Aging 2000;21: 331–42.

97. de la Torre JC. Cerebral hypoperfusion, capillary degeneration, and development of Alzheimer disease. Alzheimer Dis Assoc Disord 2000;14(Suppl 1): S72–81.

98. de la Torre JC. Alzheimer disease as a vascular disorder: nosological evidence. Stroke 2002;33:1152–62.

99. Prunell GF, Mathiesen T, Svendgaard NA. Experimental subarachnoid hemorrhage: cerebral blood flow and brain metabolism during the acute phase in three different models in the rat. Neurosurgery 2004;54:426–36 [discussion: 36–7].

100. Warkentin S, Ohlsson M, Wollmer P, et al. Regional cerebral blood flow in Alzheimer's disease: classification and analysis of heterogeneity. Dement Geriatr Cogn Disord 2004;17:207–14.

101. Johnson KA, Jones K, Holman BL, et al. Preclinical prediction of Alzheimer's disease using SPECT. Neurology 1998;50:1563–71.

102. Matsuda H. Cerebral blood flow and metabolic abnormalities in Alzheimer's disease. Ann Nucl Med 2001;15:85–92.

103. Reckelhoff JF, Romero JC. Role of oxidative stress in angiotensin-induced hypertension. Am J Physiol Regul Integr Comp Physiol 2003;284:R893–912.

104. Amouyel P, Richard F, Berr C, et al. The renin angiotensin system and Alzheimer's disease. Ann N Y Acad Sci 2000;903:437–41.

105. McKinley MJ, Albiston AL, Allen AM, et al. The brain renin-angiotensin system: location and physiological roles. Int J Biochem Cell Biol 2003;35:901–18.

106. Gard PR. The role of angiotensin II in cognition and behaviour. Eur J Pharmacol 2002;438:1–14.

107. Sharma P. Meta-analysis of the ACE gene in ischaemic stroke. J Neurol Neurosurg Psychiatr 1998;64:227–30.

108. Phillips MI, de Oliveira EM. Brain renin angiotensin in disease. J Mol Med 2008; 86:715–22.

109. Markus HS, Barley J, Lunt R, et al. Angiotensin-converting enzyme gene deletion polymorphism. A new risk factor for lacunar stroke but not carotid atheroma. Stroke 1995;26:1329–33.

110. von Bohlen und Halbach O, Albrecht D. The CNS renin-angiotensin system. Cell Tissue Res 2006;326:599–616.

111. Raghavendra V, Chopra K, Kulkarni SK. Comparative studies on the memory-enhancing actions of captopril and losartan in mice using inhibitory shock avoidance paradigm. Neuropeptides 2001;35:65–9.
112. Bonini JS, Bevilaqua LR, Zinn CG, et al. Angiotensin II disrupts inhibitory avoidance memory retrieval. Horm Behav 2006;50:308–13.
113. de Souza FA, Sanchis-Segura C, Fukada SY, et al. Intracerebroventricular effects of angiotensin II on a step-through passive avoidance task in rats. Neurobiol Learn Mem 2004;81:100–3.
114. Hu J, Igarashi A, Kamata M, et al. Angiotensin-converting enzyme degrades Alzheimer amyloid beta-peptide (A beta); retards A beta aggregation, deposition, fibril formation; and inhibits cytotoxicity. J Biol Chem 2001;276:47863–8.
115. Denny JB, Polan-Curtain J, Wayner MJ, et al. Angiotensin II blocks hippocampal long-term potentiation. Brain Res 1991;567:321–4.
116. Baranowska D, Braszko JJ, Wisniewski K. Effect of angiotensin II and vasopressin on acquisition and extinction of conditioned avoidance in rats. Psychopharmacology (Berl) 1983;81:247–51.
117. Selley ML. Increased concentrations of homocysteine and asymmetric dimethylarginine and decreased concentrations of nitric oxide in the plasma of patients with Alzheimer's disease. Neurobiol Aging 2003;24:903–7.
118. McCarron RM, Chen Y, Tomori T, et al. Endothelial-mediated regulation of cerebral microcirculation. J Physiol Pharmacol 2006;57(Suppl 11):133–44.
119. Maxwell AJ. Mechanisms of dysfunction of the nitric oxide pathway in vascular diseases. Nitric Oxide 2002;6:101–24.
120. Cooke JP, Dzau VJ. Nitric oxide synthase: role in the genesis of vascular disease. Annu Rev Med 1997;48:489–509.
121. Chen ZY, Su YL, Lau CW, et al. Endothelium-dependent contraction and direct relaxation induced by baicalein in rat mesenteric artery. Eur J Pharmacol 1999; 374:41–7.
122. Rodrigo J, Fernandez AP, Alonso D, et al. Nitric oxide in the rat cerebellum after hypoxia/ischemia. Cerebellum 2004;3:194–203.
123. Fernandez-Vizarra P, Fernandez AP, Castro-Blanco S, et al. Expression of nitric oxide system in clinically evaluated cases of Alzheimer's disease. Neurobiol Dis 2004;15:287–305.
124. Rodrigo J, Fernandez-Vizarra P, Castro-Blanco S, et al. Nitric oxide in the cerebral cortex of amyloid-precursor protein (SW) Tg2576 transgenic mice. Neuroscience 2004;128:73–89.
125. Lee TJ. Nitric oxide and the cerebral vascular function. J Biomed Sci 2000;7: 16–26.
126. Nakajima K, Uchida S, Suzuki A, et al. The effect of walking on regional blood flow and acetylcholine in the hippocampus in conscious rats. Auton Neurosci 2003;103:83–92.
127. Moro V, Kacem K, Springhetti V, et al. Microvessels isolated from brain: localization of muscarinic sites by radioligand binding and immunofluorescent techniques. J Cereb Blood Flow Metab 1995;15:1082–92.
128. Hamel E. Cholinergic modulation of the cortical microvascular bed. Prog Brain Res 2004;145:171–8.
129. Tong XK, Hamel E. Regional cholinergic denervation of cortical microvessels and nitric oxide synthase-containing neurons in Alzheimer's disease. Neuroscience 1999;92:163–75.
130. Martel CL, Mackic JB, Matsubara E, et al. Isoform-specific effects of apolipoproteins E2, E3, and E4 on cerebral capillary sequestration and blood-brain barrier

transport of circulating Alzheimer's amyloid beta. J Neurochem 1997;69: 1995–2004.

131. Rigat B, Hubert C, Alhenc-Gelas F, et al. An insertion/deletion polymorphism in the angiotensin I-converting enzyme gene accounting for half the variance of serum enzyme levels. J Clin Invest 1990;86:1343–6.

132. Alvarez R, Alvarez V, Lahoz CH, et al. Angiotensin converting enzyme and endothelial nitric oxide synthase DNA polymorphisms and late onset Alzheimer's disease. J Neurol Neurosurg Psychiatr 1999;67:733–6.

133. Monastero R, Caldarella R, Mannino M, et al. Lack of association between angiotensin converting enzyme polymorphism and sporadic Alzheimer's disease. Neurosci Lett 2002;335:147–9.

134. Lendon CL, Thaker U, Harris JM, et al. The angiotensin 1-converting enzyme insertion (I)/deletion (D) polymorphism does not influence the extent of amyloid or tau pathology in patients with sporadic Alzheimer's disease. Neurosci Lett 2002;328:314–8.

135. Bartres-Faz D, Junque C, Clemente IC, et al. Angiotensin I converting enzyme polymorphism in humans with age-associated memory impairment: relationship with cognitive performance. Neurosci Lett 2000;290:177–80.

136. Richard F, Berr C, Amant C, et al. Effect of the angiotensin I-converting enzyme I/D polymorphism on cognitive decline. The EVA Study Group. Neurobiol Aging 2000;21:75–80.

Resistant Hypertension in the Elderly

Mohammed A. Rafey, MD, MS

KEYWORDS

- Hypertension • Elderly • Pseudoresistant hypertension
- True resistant hypertension • Secondary hypertension
- Blood pressure control

Resistant hypertension is defined as "blood pressure that remains above goal in spite of the concurrent use of three antihypertensive agents of different classes. Ideally, one of the three agents should be a diuretic and all agents should be prescribed at optimal dose amounts." Recent American Heart Association guidelines also include patients who are well controlled but require four or more medications as having resistant hypertension.[1]

The Seventh Report of the Joint National Committee on Prevention, Detection, Evaluation, and Treatment of High Blood Pressure (JNC 7) recommends a goal blood pressure (BP) of less than 140/90 mm Hg in the general population, and in patients with diabetes mellitus and chronic kidney disease (CKD), a lower goal of less than 130/80 mm Hg is recommended.[2] The issue of goal BP for patients with isolated systolic hypertension, which is common in the elderly, remains a matter of debate. Clinical trials in the treatment of isolated systolic hypertension have thus far not achieved a BP goal of less than 140 mm Hg. The best evidence to date in lowering BP to less than 150 mm Hg in elderly patients is the Systolic Hypertension in the Elderly study, which showed a 38% reduction in strokes at a 10-year follow-up period.[3] However, the current consensus is a BP goal of less than 140/90 mm Hg.[2]

Resistant hypertension is prevalent across all ages but is more prevalent in elderly patients. In the Framingham study, the patient characteristic that was most strongly predictive of uncontrolled hypertension was older age; less than 25% of those older than 75 years had BP controlled to goal.[4] Data from the National Health and Nutritional Examination Survey (NHANES) also demonstrate similar results, with a much higher prevalence of uncontrolled hypertension in the older age group when compared with that in younger individuals.[5]

Although most of the data about the prevalence of resistant hypertension are derived from uncontrolled hypertension in population-based studies, the prevalence of true resistance remains uncertain. Similarly, the prognosis of true resistant hypertension remains uncertain as well, because there are no follow-up studies in this patient population.

Department of Nephrology and Hypertension, Glickman Urological and Kidney Institute, Cleveland Clinic Foundation, 9500 Euclid Avenue A-51, Cleveland, OH 44195, USA
E-mail address: rafeym@ccf.org

Clin Geriatr Med 25 (2009) 289–301
doi:10.1016/j.cger.2009.01.006
0749-0690/09/$ – see front matter © 2009 Elsevier Inc. All rights reserved.

FACTORS CAUSING RESISTANT HYPERTENSION IN THE ELDERLY

In evaluating elderly patients with resistant hypertension, it is important to first evaluate if they are truly resistant. There are several contributory reasons for the higher prevalence of uncontrolled hypertension in older individuals, including suboptimal treatment. Physician attitude toward treating elderly patients may have been influenced by the fact that the majority of hypertension trials excluded this patient group. Recently published, the Hypertension in the Very Elderly Trial (HYVET) is the first randomized, controlled trial conducted in elder hypertensive patients, and it demonstrated the benefits of antihypertensive therapy.[6] Other factors leading to inadequate therapy in the elderly include frequent side effects due to antihypertensive medications, physician fear of excessively lowering diastolic BP,[7] and patient factors, including age-related vascular hypertrophy and remodeling[8] and increased levels of sympathetic tone.[9]

Successful management of elderly patients, therefore, includes awareness, screening, and identification of contributory factors to resistant hypertension, as listed in **Table 1**.

Resistant hypertension in the elderly can thus be broadly divided into (a) false positive or Pseudoresistant hypertension and (b) true resistant hypertension.

FALSE POSITIVES OR PSEUDORESISTANT HYPERTENSION

The prevalence of false positive or pseudoresistant hypertension is higher in elderly hypertensive patients, and the most common underlying cause is pseudohypertension.

Pseudoresistance Due to Incorrect Technique in Measuring BP

Several physician- and patient-related factors have been identified that may lead to elevated BP readings in patients who are, in fact, normotensive or well controlled on antihypertensive medications. A smaller BP cuff size, rapid deflation rate of the BP cuff (a deflation rate of 2–3 mm Hg/s is generally recommended), and recent ingestion of caffeine or pressor agents are among factors that may elevate BP reading acutely at the time of measurement. The recommended method for accurate BP measurement has been described in detail in hypertension guidelines as well as in the recently released guidelines for home BP measurement.[2,10,11]

Table 1
Causes of resistant hypertension
False Positive or Pseudoresistance

• Incorrect technique in measuring BP
    • Pseudohypertension
    • Lack of adherence to lifestyle interventions
    • Foods and over-the-counter medications
    • Suboptimal therapy
    • Lack of patient adherence to antihypertensive therapy
    • White coat hypertension

True Resistant Hypertension

• Sleep apnea
    • Paroxysmal hypertension
    • Hypertension related to secondary etiology

Pseudohypertension

This is a condition in which the measured cuff pressure is inappropriately higher than true intra-arterial BP due to excessive arteriosclerosis and arterial stiffness, which is common in the elderly. Thickened and calcified arteries secondary to arteriosclerosis are not compressed adequately on inflation of the BP cuff.

Currently no reliable clinical method is available to diagnose or detect this condition. Osler's maneuver has been proposed as one of the clinical tests to identify pseudohypertension. In Osler's maneuver, the BP cuff is inflated above auscultatory systolic BP while palpating brachial or radial arterial pulses. If these arteries remain palpable despite being pulseless, then the maneuver is described as positive. Messerli and colleagues[12] demonstrated that 13 elderly patients with pseudohypertension (Osler-positive) had falsely elevated BP readings, with a difference of 10 to 54 mm Hg between cuff and intra-arterial pressure. However, later studies appear to question the reliability of Osler's maneuver.[13] Other methods of BP measurements, such as infrasonic and oscillometric techniques, have not been shown to be reliable, and intra-arterial measurement of BP remains the most definitive diagnostic test.[14]

Lack of Adherence to Recommended Lifestyle Interventions

Lifestyle interventions remain an important component in the management of hypertension at all stages. Weight reduction, smoking cessation, diet rich in fruit and vegetables patterned on the Dietary Approaches to Stop Hypertension (DASH) study, lower dietary salt intake, and regular exercise have been shown to help in lowering BP and reducing the need for additional antihypertensive medications.[15] Although hypertension guidelines generally recommend a dietary salt intake of less than 2.4 g of daily sodium intake, evidence exists that lowering this further to a daily salt intake of 1.6 mg of sodium helps in reducing the number of antihypertensive medications by at least 1 medication.[16]

Resistance to the action of diuretics and decreased efficacy of their antihypertensive effect are problems commonly noted in hypertensive patients on a higher daily intake of salt.[17] Thus, it is important to carefully evaluate the dietary history and estimate dietary salt intake in these patients.

Foods and Over-the-Counter Medications that Elevate BP

Licorice can worsen BP control by inhibiting 11 β hydroxysteroid dehydrogenase, an enzyme that increases intracellular cortisol levels and worsens hypertension.[18] There are reports that grapefruit juice can also cause elevation of BP by a similar mechanism.[19,20]

Several commonly used over-the-counter medications worsen BP control by negating the effects of antihypertensive medications. Most nonsteroidal anti-inflammatory drugs (NSAIDs) except aspirin increase sodium retention and the pressor response, thus antagonizing the effect of antihypertensive medications.[21] Sympathomimetic agents, such as pseudoephedrine and phenylpropanolamine, can raise BP.

Several other medications, as listed in **Table 2**, either (a) directly cause hypertension (eg, steroids, cyclosporine, and erythropoietin) or (b) antagonize the action of antihypertensives (eg, beta agonists such as albuterol).

Suboptimal Therapy

Suboptimal therapy is probably the most common factor that causes false-positive resistant hypertension. In the elderly, data from several studies confirm that a significant proportion of older hypertensive patients remain undertreated.[4] In the

Table 2	
Medications associated with hypertension	
• Corticotropin • Cyclosporine • Erythropoietin • Glucocorticoids • Bupropion (Wellbutrin) • Venlafaxine (Effexor) • NSAIDs	• Sympathomimetics, eg, Pseudoephedrine Phenylpropanolamine Isoproterenol Albuterol

Framingham study, among older hypertensives on treatment, 61% were receiving only one antihypertensive medication, and even fewer individuals were on a thiazide diuretic as is recommended. Randomized, controlled, prospective trials evaluating the effects of intervention with antihypertensive medications have consistently reported that optimal doses of three to four medications are generally required for improved, better BP control. Further, addition of an appropriate diuretic (either a thiazide or a loop diuretic) based on the renal function is essential for successful management of hypertension. The Antihypertensive and Lipid-Lowering Treatment to Prevent Heart Attack Trial demonstrated that the diuretic-based arm was comparable to or even superior to the non–diuretic-based arm in improving cardiovascular outcomes.[22]

Although therapeutic inertia on the part of the physician is an important factor in suboptimal therapy of hypertensive patients of all ages, additional reasons may affect decision making in the effective control of hypertension in older individuals. Most major trials evaluating antihypertensive therapy had excluded patients older than 75 years, and, as a result, until recently, there was no evidence for treating elderly patients. Further, available data derived from retrospective studies reported a shorter survival for those with systolic BP levels less than 140 mm Hg, even after adjustment for known predictors of death[23] or a significantly higher risk of death from any cause.[24] It is only recently that results from the first randomized, controlled trial, HYVET, were published, which demonstrated improved cardiovascular outcomes with optimized control of hypertension.[6]

Another important factor that may deter optimal therapy is the association of a high prevalence of hyponatremia in the elderly as a side effect of diuretics. Older women particularly appear to be at increased risk of hyponatremia.[25–28]

It is, therefore, important to use caution in treating elderly individuals with diuretics and reducing the dose to decrease side effects.[29,30] Chlorthalidone (6.25 mg) and hydrochlorthiazide (12.5 mg) are both effective diuretics with minimal side effects; a dose of 25 mg should not be exceeded for either medication.[31] An appropriate choice and dose of diuretic are crucial for effective BP control, and this is especially true in the elderly population. Loop diuretics are more efficacious than thiazides in impaired renal function with a glomerular filtration rate of less than 40 mL/min. Short-acting loop diuretics such as furosemide require frequent dosing, and higher doses are needed in CKD for efficacy and optimal BP control.[32]

Lack of Adherence to Antihypertensive Therapy

Adherence to antihypertensive therapy is known to be generally poor and may be, in fact, worse in elderly individuals.[33] Factors such as advanced age, cognitive impairment, depression, potential for adverse effects, and attitudes and beliefs have been identified as barriers to adherence and optimal BP control.[34] As hypertension is a chronic and often asymptomatic disorder, it remains a challenge for clinicians to measure, monitor, and improve adherence to prescribed therapy. Effective strategies to improve adherence include a multidisciplinary team approach incorporating patient education and ongoing support by physician and nonphysician health professionals (nurses, pharmacists, and health educators), a simplified medication regimen, and provision for self BP monitoring at home.[34,35]

White Coat Hypertension

White coat hypertension is defined as persistently elevated office BP measurements (>140/90 mm Hg) while 24-hour ambulatory BP measurements are normal and less than 135/85 mm Hg. White coat hypertension can be diagnosed with 24-hour ambulatory BP monitoring or a home BP monitor.

White coat hypertension was initially thought to be a benign condition, but recent data classify it as an entity with intermediate risk for subclinical target organ damage.[36] In a study by Polónia and colleagues,[37] patients with white coat hypertension who were followed beyond 6 years showed an increase in incidence of stroke similar to that in patients with sustained hypertension. Additional data are needed to further clarify the cardiovascular adverse effects of white coat hypertension in a more definitive manner. Based on currently available data, individuals with white coat hypertension do not appear to be at a higher risk for the development of sustained hypertension compared with that for normotensive individuals. Currently, no recommendations exist for the treatment of white coat hypertension with lifestyle interventions or antihypertensive medications.

TRUE RESISTANT HYPERTENSION

The diagnosis of true resistant hypertension should be made only after carefully excluding factors that cause false-positive resistant hypertension. In the following section, we discuss in detail some of the conditions that lead to true resistant hypertension.

Obstructive Sleep Apnea

In the elderly, the prevalence rates of obstructive sleep apnea (OSA) range from 37.5% to 62% in those older than 60 years.[38,39] Several studies have reported a strong correlation between OSA and hypertension. In a recent case-control study by Gonçalves and colleagues,[40] OSA was strongly and independently associated with resistant hypertension (odds ratio, 4.8; 95% confidence interval, 2.0–11.7). Studies in animals are the basis for several mechanisms hypothesized to explain the association between OSA and hypertension. Proposed mechanisms include chronic nighttime hypoxemia, altered chemoreceptor stimulation, and activation of sympathetic and renin-angiotensin system. Frequent nighttime hypoxia and hypercapnia also appear to stimulate aldosterone production independent of plasma renin levels.[41,42]

Treatment of OSA with noninvasive positive pressure ventilatory support in patients with hypertension appears to improve BP control.[43]

Paroxysmal Hypertension or (Pseudopheochromocytoma)

Paroxysmal hypertension or pseudopheochromocytoma is a diagnosis of exclusion. In this disorder, patients have paroxysms of hypertension associated with symptoms that are typical of pheochromocytoma, but all biochemical tests for pheochromocytoma are within normal limits.[44] Other causes such as labile hypertension or panic attacks must be ruled out. Repressed emotions secondary to emotional trauma have been hypothesized to be one of the factors in the pathogenesis of this disorder.

Management is multipronged and consists of antihypertensive medications, including beta blockers, antidepressants, and psychotherapy, which have been shown to benefit these patients.[45]

Hypertension Related to Secondary Etiology

Secondary forms of hypertension are a small fraction (less than 5%) of all hypertension. Unique disorders cause hypertension, and, in many cases, represent a curable form of hypertension. **Table 3** lists the conditions that lead to secondary hypertension.

RENAL DISORDERS
Chronic Kidney Disease

CKD is the most common cause of secondary hypertension and the second most common cause of end-stage renal disease in the United States.[46] Impaired renal function can worsen BP control by reduction in sodium and water excretion, leading to volume overload and resistant hypertension. In elderly patients, estimation of renal function by Cockcroft-Gault or Modification of Diet in Renal Disease Study (MDRD) formula is recommended, as serum creatinine level alone is not accurate.[47,48] Antihypertensive medications of choice in CKD are angiotensin-converting enzyme inhibitors and angiotensin receptor blockers. Loop diuretic alone or in combination with a thiazide-like diuretic, metolazone, may be required for good BP control.

Renovascular Disease

Fibromuscular dysplasia (FMD) and atherosclerotic renal artery disease are subtypes of renovascular disease that can cause resistant hypertension.

FMD is common in young women, whereas the atherosclerotic renal artery disease is more prevalent in elderly individuals. In a population-based study of individuals older than 65 years who underwent renal duplex ultrasound, significant stenosis was found in 6.8% of individuals.

In this study, renal artery stenosis (RAS) was independently and significantly associated with increase in age.[49] In another study evaluating causes of secondary

Table 3
Causes of secondary hypertension
Secondary Hypertension

• Renal disorders
  • Parenchymal disease
  • Renovascular disease
• Endocrine disease
  • Pheochromocytoma
  • Primary aldosteronism
  • Thyroid disease
  • Glucocorticoid excess
  • Hypercalcemia
  • Acromegaly
  • Coarctation of the aorta
• CNS tumors
• Dysautonomia
• Porphyria
• Carcinoid

Abbreviation: CNS, Central nervous system.

hypertension, increasing age and evidence of atherosclerosis were associated with a higher prevalence of RAS.[50]

Significant RAS leads to hypoperfusion of the kidney, which results in activation of renin-angiotensin-aldosterone system, leading to retention of sodium and water and worsening BP control.

Common presentations of RAS are new onset of uncontrolled hypertension or recent worsening in previously well-controlled hypertension. Patients may also present with acute worsening in renal function, asymmetric kidney size, or flash pulmonary edema, and a systolic diastolic bruit may be heard over the epigastrium.

Renal arteriogram remains the gold standard for diagnosis. Renal duplex scan, computed tomography (CT), or magnetic resonance angiogram are preferred noninvasive modalities for diagnosis, but they lack sensitivity.[51] The choice of diagnostic study should be based on available expertise in the institution where the patient is being evaluated.

Further complexity is added to the management of renovascular disease, by conflicting outcomes of studies comparing medical management with interventions, including angioplasty or renal arterial stent placement.

Medical management with antihypertensives and measures to improve atherosclerosis are the preferred modality in atherosclerotic renal artery stenosis.[52] The two main indications justifying a percutaneous intervention with angioplasty or stent placement in the elderly patients are (a) uncontrolled resistant hypertension in which the patient is at a high risk for cardiovascular and renal events and (b) acute progression of renal failure.

PRIMARY ALDOSTERONISM

Interest in the role played by aldosterone in the pathogenesis of resistant hypertension was fanned a few years ago when several studies reported elevated serum levels of aldosterone in patients with resistant hypertension.[53–55] Role of aldosterone in the pathogenesis appeared to be confirmed in a study by Nishizaka and Calhoun[56] in which they reported that addition of an aldosterone antagonist as an add-on medication in patients with resistant hypertension improved BP control even when aldosterone levels were normal. Douma and colleagues[57] recently reported that the prevalence of primary aldosteronism in patients with resistant hypertension was much lower than that previously reported. In their study of 1616 patients with resistant hypertension, 11.3% of patients were found to have aldosteronism after confirmatory salt loading test. This study was unique in applying stringent criteria for the definition of resistant hypertension and using confirmatory testing to diagnose primary aldosteronism.

A history of spontaneous hypokalemia (serum potassium of <3 mEq/L), inappropriate kaliuresis (urine potassium of >30 mEq/24 h), plasma renin activity less than 1 ng/mL/h, and plasma aldosterone greater than 22 ng/dL increases the likelihood of primary aldosteronism in a hypertensive patient. Confirmatory testing is by salt loading test, and a urinary aldosterone excretion rate greater than 14 μg/24 h in the presence of urinary sodium excretion of 250 mEq/24 h is diagnostic of primary aldosteronism.[58] Localization of tumor is done by CT scan of the adrenals. Adrenal vein sampling is performed to assess whether autonomous hormone production is unilateral or bilateral.[59]

Aldosterone plays a critical role in the regulation of potassium balance and extracellular fluid volume. Studies in animal models and humans have shown an association of elevated aldosterone levels with cardiac fibrosis.[60–62] This has been supported by studies in which addition of aldosterone antagonist improved both cardiac morbidity and mortality.[63]

Laparoscopic surgery is preferred for excision of an adrenal adenoma or unilateral hyperplasia. In patients who are not candidates for surgery or have bilateral adrenal hyperplasia, medical therapy with mineralocorticoid antagonists, such as spironolactone or epleronone, is recommended.[64]

PHEOCHROMOCYTOMA

Pheochromocytomas are chromaffin cell tumors that arise in the adrenal medulla or sympathetic ganglia and cause excess production and secretion of catecholamines. Although pheochromocytoma is often considered a disease of young and middle-aged individuals, it has been reported in the elderly population as well.[65]

Patients may present clinically with wide fluctuations in BP, sustained hypertension, or with abrupt paroxysms of hypertension. Elevations in BP may be associated with palpitations, headache, pallor, tremor, and diaphoresis. Plasma metanephrine levels have a high sensitivity and specificity in detection of pheochromocytoma.[66] Other tests include resting serum catecholamine levels and 24-hour urinary metanephrines. Since pheochromocytomas form a heterogeneous group of catecholamine-secreting tumors with variable metabolism, using multiple biochemical tests is recommended to improve accuracy in detection.[67] Imaging studies, such as CT scan and magnetic resonance imaging (MRI), have a very high sensitivity but lower specificity. A metaiodobenzylguanidine scan has a very high specificity (100%) for pheochromocytoma and is helpful when CT and MRI are inconclusive.[68] Once the tumor is identified, laparoscopic adrenalectomy is the preferred treatment of choice, and perioperative medical management of BP is the key to a successful outcome. This includes alpha blockade, preferably with selective postsynaptic alpha-1 adrenergic receptor antagonists, such as Terazocin, a calcium channel blocker for cardiac protection, and a beta blocker may be considered in case of tachyarrythmias.

MANAGEMENT OF RESISTANT HYPERTENSION

A detailed history that includes signs and symptoms, details of sodium intake, comorbid conditions, antihypertensive medication history, and history of using drugs that interfere with and increase BP levels is an essential component for initial evaluation. Accurate measurement of BP, including 24-hour ambulatory BP monitoring, may be critical in patients complaining of symptoms of orthostatic hypotension or in those with uncontrolled hypertension despite addition of antihypertensive medications in optimal doses. Physical examination should include fundoscopy to evaluate target organ damage and assessment of signs associated with secondary hypertension for example, epigastric bruit. Laboratory tests should include serum potassium, creatinine, renin, aldosterone, and plasma metanephrine levels. Estimation of renal function by calculating Cockcroft-Gault or MDRD formula is recommended. A renal duplex scan is recommended for patients with recent worsening in BP control and those at risk for atherosclerotic vascular disease. Further screening for secondary hypertension should be based on and guided by history, clinical examination, and baseline laboratory data.

TREATMENT OF RESISTANT HYPERTENSION

Lifestyle modification intervention remains the cornerstone of therapy for all types of hypertension. This includes lowering dietary salt, regular physical exercise, weight loss, and a healthy diet patterned on the DASH trial.[15]

Food and medications that interfere with hypertension therapy or cause elevation of BP should be discontinued. Antihypertensive therapy should be optimized. The choice and dose of diuretic should be individualized to each patient. If secondary hypertension is suspected, it should be thoroughly investigated, as in some instances, for example, pheochromocytoma or adrenal adenoma, this may be of curable etiology.

Noninvasive hemodynamic monitoring to individualize therapy should be considered in patients who remain resistant to treatment.[69] This involves a pathophysiological approach to treat hypertension, whereby hemodynamic parameters, such as cardiac index, systemic vascular resistance, and total body volume, are measured. Therapy is then directed to these specific physiologic parameters. For example, an increase in cardiac index is treated with a beta blocker, peripheral vascular resistance, with a vasodilator, or an increase in total body volume, with a diuretic. In a study by Taler and colleagues,[70] 104 patients with uncontrolled hypertension were randomized to a hemodynamic guided therapy or standard therapy prescribed by a specialist. At the end of 3 months, more patients in the hemodynamic guided group were controlled when compared with those in specialist care (56% versus 33%, P<.05). In a recent study, Smith and colleagues[71] reported similar results in BP control in a group of hypertensive patients who were guided by therapy directed at these abnormal hemodynamic parameters.

SUMMARY

Hypertension control has been recognized as being important in reducing cardiovascular and renal events. Clear evidence exists now that BP control in older individuals is beneficial as well. Appropriate therapy should be instituted in patients found to have a treatable cause of hypertension. In patients with resistant hypertension without an identifiable cause, noninvasive measurement of hemodynamic profile will help in instituting rational therapy targeted at abnormal hemodynamic measures to meet BP goals.

REFERENCES

1. Calhoun DA, Jones D, Textor S, et al. Resistant hypertension: diagnosis, evaluation, and treatment: a scientific statement from the American Heart Association Professional Education Committee of the Council for High Blood Pressure Research. Circulation 2008;117(25):e510–26.
2. Chobanian AV, Bakris GL, Black HR, et al. The Seventh Report of the Joint National Committee on Prevention, Detection, Evaluation, and Treatment of High Blood Pressure: the JNC 7 report. JAMA 2003;289(19):2560–72.
3. Perry HM Jr, Davis BR, Price TR, et al. Effect of treating isolated systolic hypertension on the risk of developing various types and subtypes of stroke: the Systolic Hypertension in the Elderly Program (SHEP). JAMA 2000;284:465–71.
4. Lloyd-Jones DM, Evans JC, Levy D. Hypertension in adults across the age spectrum: current outcomes and control in the community. JAMA 2005;294:466–72.
5. Franklin SS, Jacobs MJ, Wong ND, et al. Predominance of isolated systolic hypertension among middle-aged and elderly US hypertensives: analysis based on National Health and Nutrition Examination Survey (NHANES) III. Hypertension 2001;37:869–74.
6. Beckett NS, Peters R, Fletcher AE, et al. Treatment of hypertension in patients 80 years of age or older. N Engl J Med 2008;358(18):1887–98.
7. Fletcher AE, Bulpitt CJ. How far should blood pressure be lowered?. N Eng J Med 1992;326:251–4.
8. James MA, Watt PA, Potter JF, et al. Pulse pressure and resistance artery structure in the elderly. Hypertension 1995;26:301–6.

9. Grassi G. Debating sympathetic overactivity as a hallmark of human obesity: a pro's position. J Hypertens 1999;17(8):1059–60.

10. Pickering TG, Hall JE, Appel LJ, et al. Recommendations for blood pressure measurement in humans and experimental animals: Part 1: blood pressure measurement in humans: a statement for professionals from the Subcommittee of Professional and Public Education of the American Heart Association Council on High Blood Pressure Research. Hypertension 2005;45(1): 142–61.

11. Pickering TG, Miller NH, Ogedegbe G, et al. Call to action on use and reimbursement for home blood pressure monitoring: executive summary: a joint scientific statement from the American Heart Association, American Society Of Hypertension, and Preventive Cardiovascular Nurses Association. Hypertension 2008; 52(1):1–9.

12. Messerli FH, Ventura HO, Amodeo C. Osler's maneuver and pseudohypertension. N Engl J Med 1985;312(24):1548–51.

13. Wright JC, Looney SW. Prevalence of positive Osler's manoeuver in 3387 persons screened for the Systolic Hypertension in the Elderly Program (SHEP). J Hum Hypertens 1997;11:285–9.

14. Spence JD. Pseudo-hypertension in the elderly: still hazy, after all these years. Journal of Human Hypertension 1997;11:621–3.

15. Appel LJ, Moore TJ, Obarzanek E, et al. A clinical trial of the effects of dietary patterns on blood pressure. DASH Collaborative Research Group. N Engl J Med 1997;336(16):1117–24.

16. Sacks FM, Svetkey LP, Vollmer WM, et al. Effects on blood pressure of reduced dietary sodium and the Dietary Approaches to Stop Hypertension (DASH) diet. DASH-Sodium Collaborative Research Group. N Engl J Med 2001;344:3–10.

17. Wilcox CS, Loon NR, Ameer B, et al. Renal and hemodynamic responses to bumetanide in hypertension: effects of nitrendipine. Kidney Int 1989;36:719–25.

18. Walker BR, Edwards CR. Licorice-induced hypertension and syndromes of apparent mineralocorticoid excess. Endocrinol Metab Clin North Am 1994; 23(2):359–77.

19. Sardi A, Geda C, Nerici L, et al. Rhabdomyolysis and arterial hypertension caused by apparent excess of mineralocorticoids: a case report. Ann Ital Med Int 2002;17(2):126–9.

20. Lee YS, Lorenzo BJ, Koufis T, et al. Grapefruit juice and its flavonoids inhibit 11 beta-hydroxysteroid dehydrogenase. Clin Pharmacol Ther 1996;59:62–71.

21. Pope JE, Anderson JJ, Felson DT. A meta-analysis of the effects of nonsteroidal anti-inflammatory drugs on blood pressure. Arch Intern Med 1993;153(4):477–84.

22. Major outcomes in high-risk hypertensive patients randomized to angiotensin-converting enzyme inhibitor or calcium channel blocker vs diuretic: The Antihypertensive and Lipid-Lowering Treatment to Prevent Heart Attack Trial (ALLHAT). ALLHAT Officers and Coordinators for the ALLHAT Collaborative Research Group. JAMA 2002;288:2981–97.

23. Oates DJ, Berlowitz DR, Glickman ME, et al. Blood pressure and survival in the oldest old. J Am Geriatr Soc 2007;55:383–8.

24. Gueyffier F, Bulpitt C, Boissel JP, et al. Antihypertensive drugs in very old people: a subgroup meta-analysis of randomised controlled trials. INDANA Group. Lancet 1999;353:793–6.

25. Gabow PA, Moore S, Schrier RW. Spironolactone-induced hyperchloremic acidosis in cirrhosis. Ann Intern Med 1979;90:338–40.

26. Ashraf N, Locksley R, Arieff AI. Thiazide-induced hyponatremia associated with death or neurologic damage in outpatients. Am J Med 1981;70:1163–8.
27. Friedman E, Shadel M, Halkin H, et al. Thiazide-induced hyponatremia. Reproducibility by single dose rechallenge and an analysis of pathogenesis. Ann Intern Med 1989;110:24–30.
28. Sonnenblick M, Friedlander Y, Rosin AJ. Diuretic-induced severe hyponatremia. Review and analysis of 129 reported patients. Chest 1993;103:601–6.
29. Baglin A, Boulard JC, Hanslik T, et al. Metabolic adverse reactions to diuretics. Clinical relevance to elderly patients. Drug Saf 1995;12(3):161–7.
30. Salvetti A, Ghiadoni L. Thiazide diuretics in the treatment of hypertension: an update. J. Am Soc Nephrol 2006;17:S25–9.
31. Carter BL, Ernst ME, Cohen JD. Hydrochlorothiazide versus chlorthalidone: evidence supporting their interchangeability. Hypertension 2004;43:4–9.
32. Zamboli P, De Nicola L, Minutolo R, et al. Management of hypertension in chronic kidney disease. Curr Hypertens Rep 2006;8(6):497–501.
33. Lee JK, Grace KA, Taylor AJ. Effect of a pharmacy care program on medication adherence and persistence, blood pressure, and low-density lipoprotein cholesterol: a randomized controlled trial. JAMA 2006;296:2563–71.
34. Simpson RJ. Challenges for improving medication adherence. JAMA 2006; 296(21):2614–6.
35. Celis H, Den Hond E, Staessen JA. Self-measurement of blood pressure at home in the management of hypertension. Clin Med Res 2005;3(1):19–26.
36. Glen SK, Elliott HL, Curzio JL, et al. White-coat hypertension as a cause of cardiovascular dysfunction. Lancet 1996;348(9028):654–7.
37. Polónia JJ, Santos AR, Gama GM, et al. Follow-up clinic and ambulatory blood pressure in untreated white-coat hypertensive patients (evaluation after 2–5 years). Blood Press Monit 1997;2(6):289–95.
38. Ancoli-Israel S, Kripke DF, Mason W, et al. Sleep apnea and nocturnal myoclonus in a senior population. Sleep 1981;4(4):349–58.
39. Ancoli-Israel S, Kripke DF, Klauber MR, et al. Sleep-disordered breathing in community-dwelling elderly. Sleep 1991;14:486–95.
40. Gonçalves SC, Martinez D, Gus M, et al. Obstructive sleep apnea and resistant hypertension: a case-control study. Chest 2007;132:1858–62.
41. Raff H. Renin, ACTH, and aldosterone during acute hypercapnia and hypoxia in conscious rats. Am J Physiol 1988;254:R431–5.
42. Brooks D, Horner RL, Kozar LF, et al. Obstructive sleep apnea as a cause of systemic hypertension. Evidence from a canine model. J Clin Invest 1997;99: 106–9.
43. Campos-Rodriguez F, Perez-Ronchel J, Grilo-Reina A, et al. Long-term effect of continuous positive airway pressure on BP in patients with hypertension and sleep apnea. Chest 2007;132(6):1847–52.
44. Mann SJ. Severe paroxysmal hypertension (pseudopheochromocytoma): understanding the cause and treatment. Arch Intern Med 1999;159:670–4.
45. Mann SJ. Severe paroxysmal hypertension. An automatic syndrome and its relationship to repressed emotions. Psychosomatics 1996;37:444–50.
46. Foley RN, Collins A. End-stage renal disease in the United States: an update from the United States Renal Data System. J. Am Soc Nephrol 2007;18:2644–8.
47. Cockcroft DW, Gault MH. Prediction of creatinine clearance from serum creatinine. Nephron 1976;16:31–41.

48. Levey AS, Bosch JP, Lewis JB, et al. A more accurate method to estimate glomer-ular filtration rate from serum creatinine: a new prediction equation. Modification of Diet in Renal Disease Study Group. Ann Intern Med 1999;130:461–70.
49. Hansen KJ, Edwards MS, Craven TE, et al. Prevalence of renovascular disease in the elderly: a population-based study. J Vasc Surg 2002;36(3):443–5.
50. Anderson GH Jr, Blakeman N, Streeten DH, et al. The effect of age on prevalence of secondary forms of hypertension in 4429 consecutively referred patients. J Hypertens 1994;12(5):609–15.
51. Vasbinder GB, Nelemans PJ, Kessels AG, et al. Accuracy of computed tomo-graphic angiography and magnetic resonance angiography for diagnosing renal artery stenosis. Ann Intern Med 2004;114(9):674–82.
52. Tullis MJ, Caps MT, Zierler RE, et al. Blood pressure, antihypertensive medica-tion, and atherosclerotic renal artery stenosis. Am J Kidney Dis 1999;33(4): 675–81.
53. Rayner BL, Opie LH, Davidson JS. The aldosterone/renin ratio as a screening test for primary aldosteronism. S Afr Med J 2000;90:394–400.
54. Calhoun DA, Nishizaka MK, Zaman MA, et al. Hyperaldosteronism among black and white subjects with resistant hypertension. Hypertension 2002;40: 892–6.
55. Benchetrit S, Bernheim J, Podjarny E. Normokalemic hyperaldosteronism in patients with resistant hypertension. Isr Med Assoc J 2002;4:17–20.
56. Nishizaka MK, Calhoun DA. The role of aldosterone antagonists in the manage-ment of resistant hypertension. Curr Hypertens Rep 2005;7(5):343–7.
57. Douma S, Petidis K, Doumas M, et al. Revalence of primary hyperaldosteronism in resistant hypertension: a retrospective observational study. Lancet 2008; 371(9628):1921–6.
58. Bravo E. Secondary Hypertension: Mineralocorticoid Excess States. In: Black HR, Elliott WJ, editors. Hypertension: A Companion to Braunwald's Heart Disease. Philadelphia PA: Saunders Elsevier; 2007. p. 106–18.
59. Rossi GP. New concepts in adrenal vein sampling for aldosterone in the diagnosis of primary aldosteronism. Current Hypertension Reports 2007;9:90–7.
60. Brilla CG, Pick R, Tan LB, et al. Remodeling of the rat right and left ventricles in experimental hypertension. Circ Res 1990;67:1355–64.
61. González A, López B, Díez J. Fibrosis in hypertensive heart disease: role of the renin-angiotensin-aldosterone system. Med Clin N Am 2004;88:83–97.
62. Querejeta R, Varo N, López B, et al. Serum carboxy-terminal propeptide of pro-collagen type I is a marker of myocardial fibrosis in hypertensive heart disease. Circulation 2000;101:1729–35.
63. Pitt B, Zannad F, Remme WJ. The effect of spironolactone on morbidity and mortality in patients with severe heart failure. Randomized Aldactone Evaluation Study Investigators. N Engl J Med 1999;341:709–17.
64. Ghose RP, Hall PM, Bravo EL. Medical management of aldosterone-producing adenomas. Ann Intern Med 1999;131:105–8.
65. Cooper ME, Goodman D, Frauman A, et al. Phaeochromocytoma in the elderly: a poorly recognised entity? Br Med J 1986;293(6560):1474–5.
66. Lenders JW, Eisenhofer G, Mannelli M, et al. Phaeochromocytoma. Lancet 2005; 366(9486):665–75.
67. Bravo EL. Pheochromocytoma, thyroid disease, and hyperparathyroidism. J Clin Hypertens 2005;7(3):173–7.
68. Bravo EL. Pheochromocytoma: new concepts and future trends. Kidney Int 1991; 40(3):544–56.

69. Ventura HO, Taler SJ, Strobeck JE. Hypertension as a hemodynamic disease: the role of impedance cardiography in diagnostic, prognostic, and therapeutic decision making. Am J Hypertens 2005;18(2 Pt 2):26S–43S.
70. Taler SJ, Augustine J, Textor SC. Resistant hypertension: comparing hemodynamic management to specialist care. Hypertension 2002;39(5):982–8.
71. Smith RD, Levy P, Ferrario CM. Value of noninvasive hemodynamics to achieve blood pressure control in hypertensive subjects. Hypertension 2006;47(4):771–7.

Index

Note: Page numbers of article titles are in **boldface** type.

Clin Geriatr Med 25 (2009) 303–309
doi:10.1016/S0749-0690(09)00038-X
0749-0690/09/$ – see front matter © 2009 Elsevier Inc. All rights reserved.

geriatric.theclinics.com

Moving?

Make sure your subscription moves with you!

To notify us of your new address, find your **Clinics Account Number** (located on your mailing label above your name), and contact customer service at:

E-mail: elspcs@elsevier.com

800-654-2452 (subscribers in the U.S. & Canada)
314-453-7041 (subscribers outside of the U.S. & Canada)

Fax number: 314-523-5170

Elsevier Periodicals Customer Service
11830 Westline Industrial Drive
St. Louis, MO 63146

*To ensure uninterrupted delivery of your subscription, please notify us at least 4 weeks in advance of move.

ELSEVIER